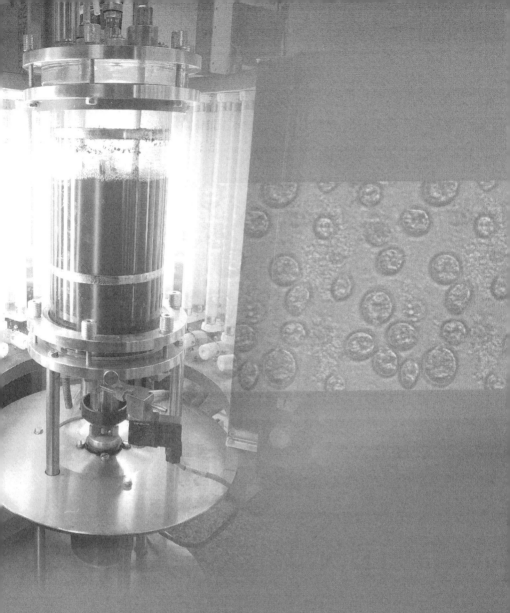

Biochemical Engineering

Biochemical Engineering
A Laboratory Manual

Debabrata Das | Debayan Das

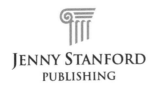

JENNY STANFORD
PUBLISHING

Published by

Jenny Stanford Publishing Pte. Ltd.
Level 34, Centennial Tower
3 Temasek Avenue
Singapore 039190

Email: editorial@jennystanford.com
Web: www.jennystanford.com

British Library Cataloguing-in-Publication Data
A catalogue record for this book is available from the British Library.

Biochemical Engineering: A Laboratory Manual

Copyright © 2021 Jenny Stanford Publishing Pte. Ltd.

ISBN 978-981-4877-36-7 (Hardcover)
ISBN 978-1-003-11105-4 (eBook)

Contents

Preface

Take risk in your life. If you win, you can lead.
If you lose, you can guide.

—Swami Vivekananda

Biochemical Engineering mostly deals with complicated life systems in comparison to Chemical Engineering. Science gives us the reasoning behind the development of a new product, whereas engineering applies the science so that the product can be manufactured at the commercial scale. The authors have recently written a book titled *Biochemical Engineering: An Introductory Textbook*, published by M/s. Jenny Stanford Publishing. The present book is an attempt to describe experimental determination of several parameters involved in the operation of a bioreactor/fermenter.

Any report writing plays a crucial role in the proper communication of facts and figures. So the book initially includes a format of laboratory report writing for the betterment of students. A fermenter/bioreactor is the heart of biochemical processes. The specialty of a fermenter is essential to operate the system under aseptic condition to allow the growth of the desired microorganisms. The metabolic pathways of microorganisms are governed by different enzymes. So the book initially discusses determination of enzymatic reaction kinetics, followed by cell growth kinetics. The operation and analysis of different biochemical processes are required to find out the special features of the same. The book also discusses in detail determination of several parameters such as maximum velocity of reaction, the Michaelis–Menten constant, maximum specific growth rate, saturation constant, true growth yield coefficient, maintenance coefficient, growth- and nongrowth-associated coefficients, air filtration efficiency, volumetric mass transfer coefficient, mixing time, determination of death rate constant, chemical oxygen demand, heat of combustion, etc.

The present book is a novel attempt to describe real experimental protocols to find out several kinetic parameters of biochemical processes as mentioned above. One of the authors has the experience of teaching Biochemical Engineering laboratory classes for more than three decades. This book is a comprehensive collection of different experiments based on the fundamentals of biochemical processes carried out by the undergraduate students of Biotechnology and Biochemical Engineering in the Indian Institute of Technology Kharagpur. It emphasizes on the determination of not only the characteristics of raw materials but also other essential parameters required for the operation of biochemical processes. It also focuses on the applicability of the analysis on different biochemical processes.

The readers will find this book a complete paraphernalia of knowledge about the experimental aspects of biochemical engineering process. Biohydrogen fermentation experimental protocol gives information on the methodology for finding out several parameters of cell growth kinetics. This information may be extended to other fermentation processes. Special experiments such as microbial fuel cells (MFCs) and biosorption kinetics are also included. The MFC is a unique devise to convert organic wastes to electricity. Contaminants (such as heavy metal ions) present in the industrial wastewater can be removed by the adsorption technique. The book consists of schematic diagrams of several experimental processes, photographs of the experimental setup, and comprehensive tables dealing with data and analysis of biochemical processes. Most of the sophisticated instruments are operated through computers. The standard operational protocols (SOPs) of a few instruments are also included at the end. Basic principles involved in the operation of different instruments have also been discussed. The proposed book is new in the market. It can be an ideal *vade mecum* for young researchers, teachers, and scientists endeavoring in the experimental aspects of biochemical engineering. The book is also appropriate for biochemical/chemical engineering, biotechnology, microbiology, and environmental biotechnology graduates, undergraduates, and industrial practitioners. Probable questions on experimental protocols have also been included at the end of the book as an exercise for self-evaluation.

The authors are thankful to Mr. Chandan Mahata and Dr. Jhansi L. Varanasi for their help in the various stages of manuscript preparation.

We hope this book will be useful to our readers!

Debabrata Das
Debayan Das
Summer 2020

List of Symbols

A_{anode}	Projected surface of anode
a_m	Surface area per unit volume
C	Cunningham's correction factors for slip flow, volume fraction of the cells in suspension, concentration
C_L	Dissolved oxygen (DO) concentration at time t
C^*	Saturated DO concentration
C_E	Coulombic efficiency
ΔC	COD removed
D	Dilution rate, impeller diameter
D_a	Damköhler number
D_{BM}	Diffusivity of the particle
d_P, d_f	Particle diameter, fiber diameter
$D_{max}, D_{washout}$	Maximum dilution rate, dilution rate for the washout of the cell
E_{An}	Anodic half-cell potential
E_{Cat}	Cathodic half-cell potential
E	Enzyme concentration at time t
e_0	Initial enzyme concentration
E_{tot}	Total open circuit voltage
F	Volumetric flow rate, Faraday constant, flow rate
g_c, g	Conversion factor, acceleration due to gravity
H_{comb}	Heat of combustion
I, I_d	Current, current density
K	Dissociation constant
k_d, k, k_1, k_2, k_{-1}	Death rate constant, reaction rate constant

k_L	Mass transfer coefficient in the liquid phase
k_a	Mass transfer coefficient
$k_L a$	Volumetric mass transfer coefficient
K_m	Michaelis–Menten constant
K_S	Saturation constant
l	Optical path length
m	Mass, maintenance coefficient
M	Amount of biomass
m_y, m_c, m_m	Mass of cells, mass of suspension, mass of media
N	Number of moles, concentration of the cells, normality
N_{Re}	Reynolds number
n	Rotational speed of the stirrer
N_S	Rate of mass transfer
N_P	Power number
N_R	Geometrical ratio
P, P_d	Product concentration, power drawn by the agitator/stirrer, power density
q_{o2}	Specific oxygen uptake by the cell
R	Gas constant, external resistance (Ω)
r_x, r_d	Rate of cell mass formation, rate of death of the cell mass
S, S_0, S_b, S_{SS}	Limiting substrate concentration, initial substrate concentration, bulk-phase substrate concentration, substrate concentration at the surface of solid matrix
T	Temperature in Kelvin
$t, t_d, t_{d,min}, t_b$	Time of reaction, doubling time, minimum doubling time, batch time
t_m	Mixing time
u	Velocity of the fluid
V, v	Volume, voltage, air velocity, rate of reaction
v_{max}, v_{obs}	Maximum velocity of enzymatic reaction, observe rate of reaction

V_p, V_R, V_C, V_m, V_y, V_{An}	Volume of the particle, volume of the reactor, critical air velocity, volume of cell suspension, volume of the medium, volume of cell, analyte volume
X	Cell mass concentration
x_0	Initial cell mass concentration
$Y_{X/S}$	Overall cell mass yield coefficient
$Y'_{X/S}$	True cell mass yield coefficient
$Y_{P/S}$	Product yield coefficient

Greek Letters

μ	Specific growth rate of the cell, viscosity
μm	Micron
μ_{max}	Maximum specific growth rate
μ_d	Specific death rate of the cell
η	Effectiveness factor, collection efficiency (experimental)
η_0	Overall collection efficiency
η_α	Single fiber efficiency
α	Growth-associated coefficient, volume fraction of the fiber
β	Nongrowth-associated coefficient
ε	Absorption coefficient
ρ	Density of the fluid
ρ_y, ρ_c, ρ_m	Density of cell, density of suspension, density of media
φ	Inertial parameter
ρ	Density of the fluid
ρ_p	Density of the particle
θ	Hydraulic retention time
ϑ	Specific product formation rate

Laboratory Report Format

Report writing is an art. The report should be written in a manner that the purpose of the experiment is well defined. This is usually presented in white data sheets or lab report book. The title page deals with the experiment number and title. The title should be short and self-explanatory. Most of the laboratory experiments are carried out by a group of students. So the names of all students must be mentioned in the cover page. This is followed by an introduction where the background of the experiment should be mentioned. This plays an important role in any report writing. So it should be carefully considered because it consists of the aims of the experiment and also the theory behind the experiment. All the mathematical equations and the nomenclatures of different parameters with the units must be mentioned. The procedure of the experiment is nothing but the work plan, which should be written in a pointwise manner. This also includes a detailed sketch of any instrument used along with its specifications and make, in case other than the custom make. A list of chemicals should also be mentioned.

The data of the experimental study must be included in the form of tables. These data are used for finding out different parameters. The sample calculations must be shown in the report. The calculated values in most of the cases must be documented in the form of tables. These calculated values are used for finding out different parameters through graphical analysis. All graphs and tables should have proper legends. The legends should explain the content of the tables and figures.

Discussions are the major portion of any experimental study because they include success of the experimental studies with respect to the reported data available in the literature. Any shortfalls of the experiment must be mentioned with proper reasoning. Your satisfaction level on any of the experimental study should be mentioned. The report-writing format of a laboratory experimental study is given in Table 1. The report should be presented as neatly as possible. The text should be written in the third person singular number.

Table 1   Report-writing format

---

1. Title page

- Experiment number and title
- Name and date
- Class, section, and group (including names)

2. Introduction

- Background statement (if necessary)
- Why did you do the experiment (objective)?
- Theory behind experiment (including any equations used)

3. Procedure

- How did you do the experiment?
- Equipment used
- Sketch of equipment (with dimensions)

4. Calculations

- Sample or complete
- Show formulas used and explain terms
- State units used

5. Results

- Tabular form whenever possible (with units)
- Graphical form when helpful (plotted on proper graph paper with title, units, and your name)

6. Discussion

- Validity of results (comparison with accepted values or theory)
- Percentage of error
- Sources of error

7. Calculations

- Implications of results
- Value of experiment (personal opinion)

8. Data sheet and handout material

- Original data sheet(s) must be included.
- For an informal report, points 2, 3, and 7 may be left out. The report should be written neatly on a plain white paper or engineering paper. Be concise and brief; write in the third person singular.
- Tense. Communication is the name of the game.

Experiment 1

Layout of a Fermenter with Controller

Objective: To identify different parts of the fermenter

1.1 Introduction

A fermenter is a vessel that maintains aseptic conditions of the medium with proper composition for the growth of desirable microorganisms. It is used in both the laboratory and the industry for the commercial production of oxychemicals, antibiotics, hormones, etc. The main function of a fermenter is to provide optimized conditions for the growth of a pure culture or a defined mixture of microorganisms or animal cells to obtain the desired product.

Different types of fermenters have been designed till date based on their application in different areas of research and industrial processes. The fermentation process is carried out in a strict sceptic condition. So, while constructing a fermenter, the selection of materials plays an especially important role. The material of construction of a fermenter is usually stainless steel, like SS316 (Fig. 1.1).

Fermenter type: KLF2000

Make of the fermenter: BIOENGINEERING AG Sagenrainstrasse7 CH-8636 Wald.

Biochemical Engineering: A Laboratory Manual
Debabrata Das and Debayan Das
Copyright © 2021 Jenny Stanford Publishing Pte. Ltd.
ISBN 978-981-4877-36-7 (Hardcover), 978-1-003-11105-4 (eBook)
www.jennystanford.com

1.2 Accessories of Fermenter

1.2.1 Aeration System

The primary purpose of the aeration system is to provide micro-organisms in the submerged culture with sufficient oxygen for metabolic requirements. This comprises the following:

(i) *Compressor*: A compressor is a mechanical device that increases the pressure of air by reducing its volume and forces more and more gas in the storage tank. It should be free from particulate matters and oil in the air.

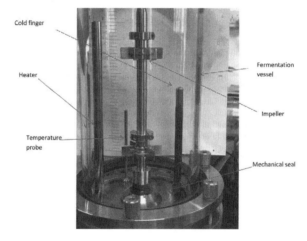

Figure 1.1   Different parts of the fermenter.

(ii) *Rotameter*: A rotameter is a device that measures the flow rate of fluid in a closed tube by allowing variation in the cross-sectional area the fluid travels through, causing a measurable effect. It has a linear vertical scale (Fig. 1.2).

(iii) *Air filter*: An air filter is a device composed of fibrous materials (hollow fiber membranes, HFMs), which removes solid particulars such as dust pollen, mold, and bacteria from air. HFMs are a class of artificial membranes containing a semipermeable barrier in the form of a hollow fiber (Fig. 1.3).

(iv) *Non-return valve*: A non-return valve is a one-way valve that normally allows fluid to flow through it in only one direction.

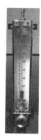

Figure 1.2 Rotameter.

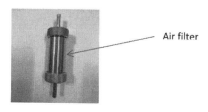

Figure 1.3 Air filter.

The purpose of the valve is to prevent the accidental reverse flow of liquid or gas in a pipe due to the breakdown of the pump or power supply (Fig. 1.4).

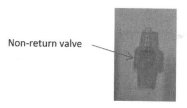

Figure 1.4 Non-return valve.

1.2.2 Mechanical Seal

The mechanical seal consists of two parts: The stationary part is the bearing and the other part is the rotation shaft. The two components are pressed together by springs and packaging materials. In the industrial fermentation process, a sterilized antifoam oil lubricates the shaft. Antifoam is passed through a chiller for cooling.

1.2.3 Fermenter Vessel

For small-scale fermentation, both glass and stainless vessels are used. The volume of a lab fermentation vessel is 3.4 L. Glass vessels are usually smooth, and this smoothness makes them nontoxic and corrosion proof. It is easy to examine the interior of the vessel. These vessels may be sterilized in vitro or in situ. In vitro sterilization is carried out in an autoclave, whereas in situ sterilization is done with the help of an electrical heater or live steam without the movement of the vessel.

1.2.4 Feed Ports

Feed ports are silicon tubes connected to the nutrient reservoir. They are used to add nutrients and other important substituents in the fermenter vessel.

1.2.5 Baffles

Baffles are metal strips attached radially to the wall of the fermenter. They are used to prevent vortex and to improve aeration capacity (oxygen transfer efficiency). Baffles maintain a gap between them and the vessel wall to enable scouring action, thus minimizing microbial growth on the walls of the fermenter (Fig. 1.5).

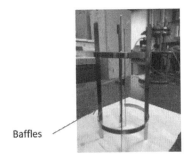

Baffles

Figure 1.5   Baffles of the fermenter.

1.2.6 Impeller

An impeller is used for mechanical agitation, which is required to ensure that a uniform suspension of microbial cells is achieved in a homogeneous nutrient medium.

1.2.7 Sparger

A sparger is used for aeration. The purpose of aeration is to provide sufficient oxygen to the microorganism for metabolic requirements. A sparger introduces air into the liquid in the vessel. It can be of three types: porous, orifice, and nozzle.

1.2.8 Outlet

Reflux cooler: The air flowing out of the fermenter has the same temperature as that during cultivation and is also correspondingly saturated. The moisture is condensed out with a reflux cooler, and then the condensate is returned to the fermenter. This helps to keep the liquid volume of the fermenter constant.

Exhaust air filter: It is used to filter the air going out of the fermenter to prevent environmental pollution. During power cut, the air inlets are closed, and then the exhaust air filter supplies filtered air required for the survival of cells.

Outlet valve: It regulates the release of air or liquid from the fermenter.

1.2.9 Safety Valve

Safety valves ensure that the pressure never exceeds the safe upper limit of the specified value to avoid explosion.

1.3 Temperature Loop

1.3.1 Heater

Heat is generally provided to the fermenter by internal coils, which get heated up and directly heat the medium. A thermostatically controlled water bath can also be used.

1.3.2 Cold Finger

A cold finger is a closed coil or pipe in which the coolant liquid (cold water, etc.) can enter and exit. It is used to generate generalized cooling.

1.3.3 Solenoid Valve

A solenoid valve is an electrically controlled valve used for maintaining the temperature of the fermentation broth (Fig. 1.6).

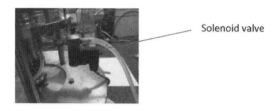

Solenoid valve

Figure 1.6 Electrically control solenoid valve.

1.4 Monitoring and Control Loop

1.4.1 Temperature Probe

A temperature probe is used to measure the temperature of the culture broth in the **(Pt 100)** fermenter vessel. It is known as a thermostat, which is electrically controlled. This sensor is usually made of bimetals.

1.4.2 pH Probe

A pH probe is used to monitor the pH of the culture broth during the growth of microbes and reaction in the vessel (Figs. 1.8–1.10). It is known as a sterilizable pH probe (Das and Das, 2019) because it can withstand the high steam pressure (15 psi) of the fermenter during

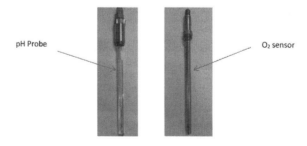

pH Probe

O$_2$ sensor

Figure 1.7 pH and dissolved oxygen probes of the fermenter.

in situ sterilization of the medium. This pressure is maintained on the surface of the electrolyte present in the pH probe with the help of a hand pump. These probes are manufactured by Mettler Toledo, Ingold, etc. A pH probe is calibrated using standard pH buffer solution (Fig. 1.7).

1.4.3 O_2 Sensor

An O_2 sensor monitors the dissolved oxygen concentration of the fermentation broth. These sensors are manufactured by Mettler Toledo. An O_2 sensor is calibrated by sparging nitrogen and air separately.

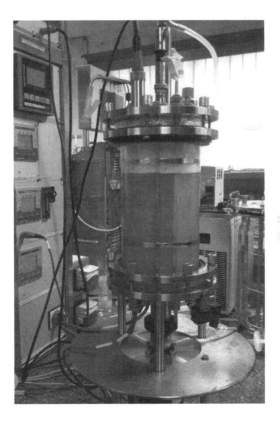

Figure 1.8 Bioengineering AG fermenter, Switzerland.

1.4.4 Motor

A motor provides energy to the impeller to stir the culture medium. It can be either bottom driven or top driven.

1.5 Peristaltic Pump

A peristaltic pump is used for the aseptic transfer of the medium to the fermenter. The basic principle is the compression and relaxation of the tubing connected with the feed tank. The medium remains

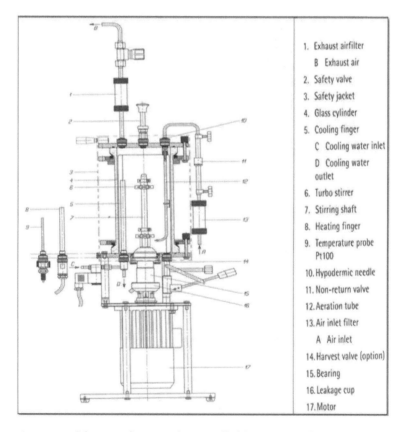

1. Exhaust airfilter
   B Exhaust air
2. Safety valve
3. Safety jacket
4. Glass cylinder
5. Cooling finger
   C Cooling water inlet
   D Cooling water outlet
6. Turbo stirrer
7. Stirring shaft
8. Heating finger
9. Temperature probe Pt100
10. Hypodermic needle
11. Non-return valve
12. Aeration tube
13. Air inlet filter
    A Air inlet
14. Harvest valve (option)
15. Bearing
16. Leakage cup
17. Motor

Figure 1.9   Schematic diagram of a controlled fermenter and its accessories.

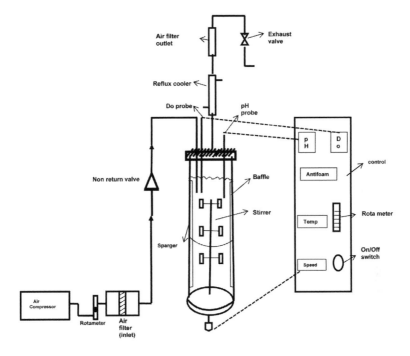

Figure 1.10   Schematic diagram on the operation of the fermenter.

inside a flexible silicon tube. The companies supplying this pump are Watson Marlow, Cole Parmer, etc.

1.6 Foam Control

A probe (foam sensing and control unit) is inserted through the top plate. It is set at a defined level above the broth surface. When the foam rises and touches the probe surface/tip, a current is passed through the circuit, which actuates the pump, and an antifoam is released within seconds to the fermentation vessel. The pump is switched off as soon as the foam subsides.

Experiment 2

Enzymatic Reaction Kinetics

Objective: To determine K_m and v_{max} of starch hydrolysis by alpha-amylase

2.1 Enzyme Activity

Enzyme activity indicates catalytic ability. It can be measured by two methods: by measuring the decrease in substrate concentration in a period of time and by measuring the increase in the concentration of a product after a period of time. The catalytic activity of an enzyme can be expressed in international units (expressed as IU): 1 IU/mL (μmol/min mL) is defined as the amount of enzyme that catalyzes the conversion of 1 μmol of substrate degraded or product formed per minute per mL of enzymatic solution under the specified conditions of the assay method.

2.1.1 Alpha-Amylase Activity

Alpha-amylase (α-amylase) is an enzyme EC 3.2.1.1 that hydrolyzes alpha bonds of large, alpha-linked polysaccharides, such as starch and glycogen, yielding glucose and maltose. It is the major form

Biochemical Engineering: A Laboratory Manual
Debabrata Das and Debayan Das
Copyright © 2021 Jenny Stanford Publishing Pte. Ltd.
ISBN 978-981-4877-36-7 (Hardcover), 978-1-003-11105-4 (eBook)
www.jennystanford.com

of amylase found in humans and other mammals. It is used for the degradation of starch for ethanol production by *Saccharomyces cerevisiae.*

2.2 Enzymatic Reaction Kinetics

For the following simple homogeneous reaction,

$$S \xrightarrow{E} P$$

the reaction rate may be expressed as

$$V = -\frac{ds}{dt} = \frac{dp}{dt}$$

where S, P are the molar concentration of substrate and product, respectively; v is the velocity of reaction; and E is the enzyme.

A typical experiment to determine the enzyme kinetics parameters might proceed as follows: At time zero, solutions of substrate and an appropriate purified enzyme are mixed in a well-stirred, closed isothermal vessel containing a buffer solution to control pH. The substrate and/or product concentrations are monitored at various later times. The substrate degradation and product formation profiles are shown in Fig. 2.1.

The reproducibility of an enzymatic activity plays an important role in the reactor design of an isolated enzyme. Enzymes can loss their activity due to denaturation and other environmental factors. The enzymatic reaction kinetics equation was proposed by Leonor Michaelis and Maud Menten.

2.2.1 Michaelis–Menten Kinetics

The relationship between the substrate concentration and the velocity of the enzymatic reaction can be represented by the Michaelis–Menten equation as follows:

$$v = \frac{v_{max}S}{K_m + s} \tag{2.1}$$

where v is the velocity of reaction, moles/(vol)(time); v_{max} is the maximum velocity of reaction, moles/(vol)(time); S is the substrate

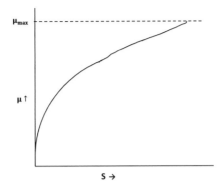

Figure 2.1   Relationship between the velocity of reaction and the substrate concentration.

concentration, moles/vol; K_m is the Michaelis–Menten constant, moles/vol.

Equation 2.1 has been proposed on the basis of the relationship between v and S as shown in Fig. 2.1. The qualitative features of Eq. 2.1 and Fig. 2.1 are as follows:

- At low substrate concentration, the order of the reaction follows first-order kinetics.
- At high substrate concentration, it follows zero-order kinetics.
- The maximum velocity of the reaction is directly proportional to the total enzyme concentration as shown below:

$$v_{max} \rightarrow ke_0 \qquad (2.2)$$

where k is the reaction rate constant and e_o is the total enzyme concentration.

George Briggs and J.B.S. Haldane justified Eq. 2.1 by considering the following reaction pattern (Eq. 2.3 and Eq. 2.4), which is based on loosely binding the substrate on the active site of the enzyme molecule and then it gives the product.

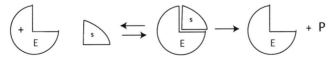

The overall reaction can be expressed as follows:

$$E + S \leftrightarrow ES \rightarrow P + E \qquad (2.3)$$

The above reaction can represented as

$$E + S \frac{k_1}{k_1} ES \rightarrow k_2 E + p \qquad (2.4)$$

The velocity of the above reaction may be written as follows:

$$v = -\frac{ds}{dt} = k_1 \lfloor S \rfloor [E] - k_1 [Es] \qquad (2.5)$$

and

$$\frac{d\lceil Es \rceil}{dt} = k_1 [E][S] - (k_1 + k_2)ES \qquad (2.6)$$

The quasi-steady state condition is such that the reaction is assumed to be in a steady state, which can be validated for the present case provided the small. At such condition

$$\frac{d\,[ES]}{dt} = 0 \qquad (2.7)$$

Again

$$[E]_o = [E] + [ES]$$

or

$$[E] = [E]_o - [ES] \qquad (2.8)$$

Equation 2.6 can be written as

$$k_1\,[E]\,[S] - (k_{-1} + k_2)\,[ES] = 0 \qquad (2.9)$$

Putting the value of $[E]$ from Eq. 2.8, we get

$$k_1\,([E]_o - [ES])\,[S] - (k_{-1} + k_2)\,[ES] = 0 \qquad (2.10)$$

or

$$k_1\,[E]_o\,[S] - [ES]\,(k_1\,[S] + (k_{-1} + k_2)) = 0$$

or

$$[ES] = \frac{K_1\,[E]_o\,[S]}{K_1\,[S] + K_{-1} + K_2} \qquad (2.11)$$

Again, from Eq. 2.5, we get

$$v = k_1\,[S]\,[E]_o - [ES]\,(k_1\,[S] + k_{-1}) \qquad (2.12)$$

Substituting the $[ES]$ from Eq. 2.11, we get

$$v = k_1 [S] [E]_0 - \frac{k_1 [E]_0 [S] (k_1 [S] + k_{-1})}{k_1 [S] + k_{-1} + k_2}$$

$$= k_1 [S] [E]_0 \left[1 - \frac{k_1 [S] + k_{-1}}{k_1 [S] + k_2 + k_{-1}} \right]$$

$$= \frac{k_1 k_2 [S] [E]_0}{k_1 [S] + k_2 + k_{-1}}$$

$$= \frac{k_2 [E]_0 [S]}{\frac{k_2 + k_{-1}}{k} + [S]} = \frac{v_{max} [S]}{K_m + [S]} \tag{2.13}$$

where $k_2 [E]_0 = v_{max}$ and $\frac{k_2 + k_{-1}}{k_1} = K_m$. The Michaelis constant K_m is an inverse measure of the strength of substrate binding.

It is assumed that the first-step of reaction between enzyme and substrate is reversible and at equilibrium condition rate of forward reaction is equal to rate of backward reaction. This may be represented as follows

$$\frac{[S] [E]}{[ES]} = \frac{k_{-1}}{k_1} = K = \text{dissociation constant}$$

The concentration profiles of different components present in the above reaction mixture are shown in Fig. 2.2.

Again, the time course of the reaction can be determined analytically by integrating Eq. 2.13 as follows

$$v = -\frac{ds}{dt} + \frac{V_{max} S}{K_m + s}$$

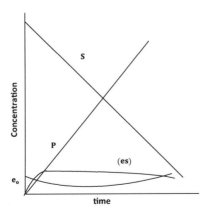

Figure 2.2 Concentration profiles of the different components present in the reaction.

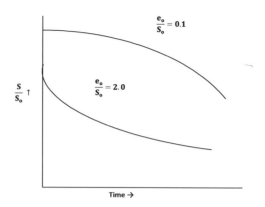

Figure 2.3 Correlation of substrate concentration profiles with respect to change in $\frac{e_0}{S_0}$.

or

$$-\left(K_m \int_{S_0}^{S} d\ln + \int_{S_0}^{S} ds \right) = v_{\max} \int_{0}^{t} dt \qquad (2.14)$$

Assume that at time $t = 0$, substrate concentration $= S_0$.
   At time t, substrate concentration $= S$.

$$K_m \ln \frac{S_0}{S} + (S_0 - S) = v_{\max}\, t \qquad (2.15)$$

Equation 2.15 can be used to find out the substrate concentration after the time t.

2.2.2 Limitation of the Michaelis–Menten Equation

Figure 2.3 reveals that the deviation from the quasi-steady state approximation is significant when the total enzyme concentration approaches. Consequently, the Michaelis–Menten equation should not really be used in such cases [3, 4].

2.2.3 Determination of Kinetic Constants

Kinetics parameters such as $v_{\max}$ and K_m can be determined from the following equations derived from Eq. 2.13:

$$\frac{1}{v} = \frac{1}{v_{\max}} + \frac{K_m}{v_{\max}} \frac{1}{S} \qquad (2.16)$$

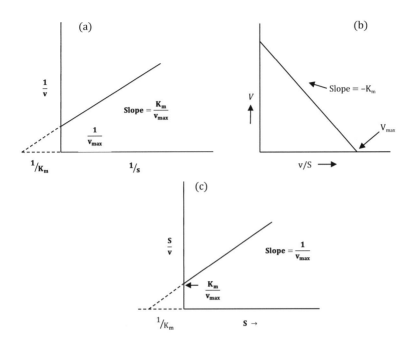

Figure 2.4 Estimation of different kinetics parameters by using different plots: (a) Lineweaver–Burk plot, (b) Eadie–Hofstee plot, and (3) Hanes–Woolf plot.

$$v = v_{\text{max}} - K_{\text{m}} \frac{v}{S} \qquad (2.17)$$

$$\frac{S}{v} = \frac{K_{\text{m}}}{v_{\text{max}}} + \frac{1}{v_{\text{max}}} S \qquad (2.18)$$

The kinetic parameters can be estimated by using several plots like

(1) Correlation of $1/v$ versus $1/S$ is known as the Lineweaver–Burk plot.
(2) Correlation of v versus v/S is known as the Eadie–Hofstee plot.
(3) Correlation of S/v versus S is known as the Hanes–Woolf plot.

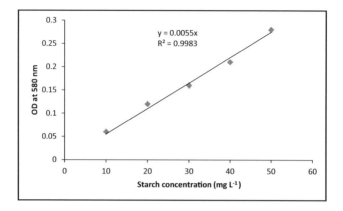

Figure 2.5   Calibration curve of starch solution.

2.3 Calibration Curve of the Substrate

Starch is used as substrate in the reaction with α-amylase. Starch is estimated by the starch–iodine method described by Xiao et al. [1]. The estimation procedure is mentioned below:

(1) Take 40 µL of starch solution in a clean microplate.
(2) Add 20 µL of 1 M HCl to stop enzymatic reaction in the microplate.
(3) Pour 100 µL of iodine reagent (5 mM I_2 and 5 mM KI) in the plate.
(4) Measure the absorbance of the developed color (dark blue) at 580 nm using a UV-VIS spectrophotometer.

2.4 Preparation of Enzyme Solution

Freeze-dried α-amylase was added to 0.1 M sodium phosphate buffer (pH 7.0) to the concentration of 1 mg/mL. This enzyme stock solution was stored at 4°C for future tests.

2.4.1 Procedure

(1) Prepare different concentrations of soluble starch concentration in five test tubes (2 to 10 g/L).

(2) Ensure 9 mL of starch solution in a test tube.
(3) Add 1 mL of enzyme solution.
(4) Keep the mixtures in an incubator shaker for 10 min at 37°C.
(5) Analyze the sample for the estimation of residual starch.

2.5 Observation

Table 2.1 Starch concentration after the enzymatic reaction

Initial bulk starch concentration (g/L)	Final bulk starch concentration (g/L)
10	7.126
8	5.183
6	3.297
4	1.518
2	0.054

2.6 Results

Kinetic parameters such as K_m and v_{max} were determined using the reciprocal of the Michaelis–Menten equation, i.e., the Lineweaver–Burk plot [2].

$$\frac{1}{v} = \frac{K_m}{v_{max}} \frac{1}{S_0} + \frac{1}{v_{max}}$$

where v is the rate of reaction at the particular starch concentration.

Table 2.2 Calculated data

Initial starch concentration (S_0) (g/L)	Final starch concentration (S) (g/L)	Rate of reaction (v) (g/L min)	$1/S_0$	$1/v$
10	7.126	0.287	0.1	3.48
8	5.183	0.282	0.125	3.55
6	3.297	0.270	0.16	3.7
4	1.518	0.248	0.25	4.03
2	0.054	0.194	0.5	5.14

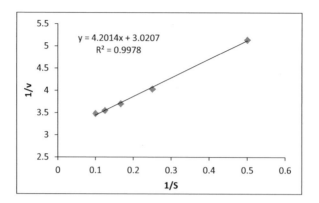

Figure 2.6 Lineweaver–Burk plot.

From Fig. 2.6, we get $v_{max} = 0.331$ g/L min and $K_m = 1.391$ g/L.

2.6.1 Sample Calculations

From Fig. 2.6, we get slope $= 4.2014 = \frac{K_m}{v_{max}}$, intercept $= 3.0207 = \frac{1}{v_{max}}$.

So $v_{max} = 0.331$g/L min, $K_m = 4.2014 \times 0.331 = 1.391$g/L.

2.7 Discussion

The kinetic constants v_{max} and K_m of the enzyme indicate the suitability of the enzyme for product formation. Higher values of v_{max} and lower values of K_m increase the enzymatic reaction significantly. However, a higher value of K_m signifies a higher amount of substrate requirement as compared to that of lower value for the same amount of product formation.

References

1. Xiao, Z., Storms, R., and Tsang, A., A quantitative starch–iodine method for measuring alpha-amylase and glucoamylase activity, *Analytical Chemistry*, **351**: 146–148, 2006.

2. Das, D. and Das, D., *Biochemical Engineering: An Introductory Textbook*, Jenny Stanford Publishing, 2019.

3. Bailey, J. E. and Ollis, D. F. *Biochemical Engineering Fundamentals*, McGraw-Hill Inc., New Delhi, India, 2010.

4. Doran, P. M. *Bioprocess Engineering Principles*, Second Edition, Academic Press, Waltham, USA, 2012.

Experiment 3

Kinetics of the Immobilized Enzymatic Reaction

Objective: To determine K_m and v_{max} of starch hydrolysis by immobilized α-amylase using external mass transfer diffusion

3.1 Preparation of Enzyme Solution

Freeze-dried α-amylase (EC 3.2.1.1) is added to 0.1 M sodium phosphate buffer (pH 7.0) to the concentration of 1 mg/mL. This enzyme stock solution was stored at 4°C for future tests.

3.1.1 Definition of Enzyme Immobilization

Immobilized enzymes are defined as confinement or localization of the enzymes in a certain defined region of space of an inert, insoluble material with retention of their catalytic activities, which can be reused again and again in a continuous mode of operation.

3.2 Kinetic Theory

The diffusional problem of the substrate using an immobilized enzyme plays an important role. It is classified as (a) external mass

Biochemical Engineering: A Laboratory Manual
Debabrata Das and Debayan Das
Copyright © 2021 Jenny Stanford Publishing Pte. Ltd.
ISBN 978-981-4877-36-7 (Hardcover), 978-1-003-11105-4 (eBook)
www.jennystanford.com

transfer resistance and (b) internal mass transfer resistance. The external mass transfer resistance has been taken into consideration in the present experimental study to find out the kinetics of the immobilized enzyme.

In case the enzyme is immobilized only on the external surface of the solid matrix, then mass transport is to be considered from the bulk solution to the surface of the solid matrix and reaction occurs at that position. This is known as the external mass transfer resistance.

The rate of mass transfer from the bulk solution to a surface,

$$N_S = k_a a_m (S_b - S_S) \tag{3.1}$$

where k_a is the mass transfer coefficient, a_m is the surface area per unit volume, S_b is the bulk-phase substrate concentration, and S_S is the substrate concentration at the surface of the solid matrix.

The Michaelis–Menten equation may be written as

$$v = \frac{v_{max} S_S}{K_m + S_S} \tag{3.2}$$

At steady-state (SS) conditions,

Mass transfer rate = Rate of reaction at the surface of the solid matrix

where internal diffusion limitations are not significant.

So at SS condition, we can write from Eq. 3.1 and Eq. 3.2 as

$$k_a a_m (S_b - S_s) = \frac{v_{max} S_s}{K_m + S_s} = v \tag{3.3}$$

$$\therefore S_s = S_b - \frac{v}{k_a a_m} = \frac{(S_b k_a a_m - v)}{k_a a_m} \tag{3.4}$$

Equation 3.2 may be written as

$$\frac{1}{v} = \frac{1}{v_{max}} + \frac{K_m}{v_{max}} \frac{1}{S_s} \tag{3.5}$$

Putting the value of S_s from Eq. 3.4 in Eq. 3.2, we get

$$\frac{1}{v} = \frac{1}{v_{max}} + \frac{K_m}{v_{max}} \frac{k_a a_m}{(S_b k_a a_m - v)} \tag{3.6}$$

$$\frac{1}{v} = \frac{1}{v_{max}} + \frac{K_m}{v_{max}} \frac{1}{S_b} \frac{k_a a_m}{\left(k_a a_m - \frac{v}{S_b}\right)} \tag{3.7}$$

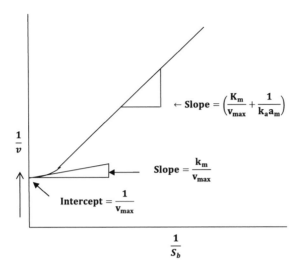

Figure 3.1 Plot of $1/v$ versus $1/S_b$ using immobilized enzyme.

$$\frac{1}{v} = \frac{1}{v_{max}(S_b k_a a_m - v)}(S_b k_a a_m - v + K_m a_m k_a)$$

$$\frac{S_b k_a a_m}{v} - \frac{v}{v} = \frac{1}{v_{max}}(S_b k_a a_m + K_m a_m k_a - v)$$

$$\frac{S_b k_a a_m v_{max}}{v} = S_b k_a a_m + K_m a_m k_a - v + v_{max}$$

$$\frac{1}{v} = \frac{1}{S_b}[S_b k_a a_m + K_m a_m k_a - v + v_{max}]\frac{1}{k_a a_m v_{max}}$$

$$\frac{1}{v} = \frac{1}{S_b}\left[\frac{S_b}{v_{max}} + \frac{K_m}{v_{max}} - \frac{v}{k_a a_m v_{max}} + \frac{1}{k_a a_m}\right] \qquad (3.8)$$

The plot $\frac{1}{v}$ versus $\frac{1}{S_b}$ is shown in Fig. 3.5.

Again Eq. 3.7 may be written as

$$\left[\frac{1}{v} = \frac{1}{v_{max}} + \left(\frac{K_m}{v_{max}}\right)\left(\frac{1}{S_b}\right)\frac{1}{\left(1 - \frac{v}{S_b k_a a_m}\right)}\right] \qquad (3.9)$$

When $S_b \to \alpha$, i.e., at $\frac{1}{S_b} \to 0$, in Fig. 3.1, Slope $= \frac{K_m}{v_{max}}$, Intercept $= \frac{1}{v_{max}}$.

Again, when $S_b \rightarrow 0$, Eq. 3.8 may be written as

$$\frac{1}{v} = \frac{1}{S_b} \left(\frac{K_m}{v_{max}} + \frac{1}{k_a a_m} \right) \tag{3.10}$$

In Fig. 3.1, when $\frac{1}{S_b} \rightarrow \alpha$,

the slope of the straight line $= \left(\frac{K_m}{v_{max}} + \frac{1}{k_m a_m} \right)$.

So the values of K_m, v_{max}, and $k_a a_m$ can be determined from Fig. 3.1, which are the reaction kinetics parameters of the immobilized enzyme system [1, 3, 4].

3.2.1 Effectiveness Factor and Damköhler Number

The influence of mass transfer on the overall reaction process is expressed using the effectiveness factor (η) as follows

$$\eta = \frac{\text{Observed rate of reaction}}{\text{Rate of reaction in case of no mass transfer resistance, i.e. } S_s = S_b} \tag{3.11}$$

The Michaelis–Menten equation may be written as

$$\text{Observed reaction rate } (v_{obs}) = \frac{v_{max} S_s}{K_m + S_s} \tag{3.12}$$

The reaction rate with no mass transfer limitation

$$(v_{S_s \rightarrow S_b}) = \frac{v_{max} S_b}{K_m + S_b} \tag{3.13}$$

$$\eta = \frac{v_{obs}}{v_{S_s \rightarrow S_b}}$$

$$\eta = \frac{v_{max} S_s (K_m + S_b)}{(K_m + S_s) v_{max} S_b}$$

$$\eta = \frac{S_s (K_m + S_b)}{S_b (K_m + S_s)} \tag{3.14}$$

$$\text{Putting, } x = \frac{S_s}{S_b}, \quad K = \frac{K_m}{S_b}$$

$$\eta = \frac{x/(k+x)}{1/(k+1)} = \frac{x(k+1)}{(k+x)} \tag{3.15}$$

The Damköhler number (Da) is a dimensionless number and may be represented as

$$Da = \frac{\text{Maximum rate of reaction}}{\text{Maximum rate of mass transfer}} = \frac{v_{max}}{k_a a_m S_b} \quad (3.16)$$

$\eta < 1$ indicates the effect of increasing mass transfer resistance and reduction in observed activity.

Under the SS condition from Eq. 3.3,

$$k_a a_m (S_b + S_s) = \frac{v_{max} S_s}{K_m + S_s}$$

$$k_a a_m S_b \left(1 - \frac{S_s}{S_b}\right) = \frac{v_{max} \frac{S_s}{S_b}}{\frac{K_m}{S_b} + \frac{S_s}{S_b}}$$

$$\frac{v_{max}}{Da}(1-x) = \frac{v_{max}}{k+x}$$

$$\frac{1-x}{Da} = \frac{x}{K+x} \quad (3.17)$$

$$\eta = \frac{v_{obs}}{v_{Ss \to S_b}} = \frac{\frac{v_{max} S_s}{K_m + S_s}}{\frac{v_{max} S_b}{K_m + S_s}} = \frac{\frac{\frac{S_s}{S_b}}{\frac{K_m}{S_b} + \frac{S_s}{S_b}}}{\frac{S_b}{\frac{K_m}{S_b} + \frac{S_s}{S_b}}} = \frac{\frac{x}{k+x}}{\frac{1}{k+1}} = \frac{x(k+1)}{k+x} \quad (3.18)$$

From Eq. 3.17 and Eq. 3.18,

$$\frac{1-x}{Da} = \frac{\eta}{k+1} \quad (3.19)$$

$$\eta = \frac{x}{(K+x)}(k+1) = \frac{(1-x)(K+1)}{Da} \quad (3.20)$$

Equation 3.20 is the correlation between Da and η

3.2.1.1 Determination of the factor affects overall rate of the reaction

In case $Da \to 0$ (very slow rate of reaction as compared to maximum mass transfer), $x \to 1$, and then from Eq. 3.15, $\eta = 1$. Here the observed reaction kinetics is the same as the true intrinsic kinetics at the fluid–solid interface. So the reaction kinetics may be represented as

$$\bar{v} = \frac{v_{max} S_b}{K_m + S_b} \qquad (3.21)$$

Again, from Eq. 3.17, the substrate mass balance becomes

$$\frac{1-x}{Da} = \frac{x}{K + x}$$

where $0 \le x \le 1.0$

The diffusion-limited regime of system with coupling between chemical reaction and mass transfer arises when v_{max} is much larger than $k_a a_m S_b$.

When $Da \gg 1$ and x approaches zero, Eq. 3.19 becomes

$$\eta = \frac{1+k}{Da}$$

So the reaction kinetics may be represented as

$$\bar{v} = k_m a_m S_b \qquad (3.22)$$

Hence, so long as Da is very large, the observed rate of reaction $\bar{v}$ is first order with respect to bulk substrate concentration and is independent of the intrinsic rate parameters v_{max} and K_m.

3.3 Preparation of Immobilized Enzyme

A 3.5% w/v sodium alginate solution in 50 mM sodium phosphate buffer (pH 7.0) is prepared by warming at 50°C. After cooling down to room temperature, 1 mL of enzyme stock solution is mixed with 9 mL of sodium alginate solution (the total volume of the matrix and the enzyme mixture being 10 mL). The mixture is taken in a syringe, and beads are formed by dropping the solution into 1 M calcium chloride solution with gentle stirring at 4°C for 2 h. The formed beads are recovered by filtration and thoroughly washed with distilled water. The beads are dried using a filter paper (Whatman no. 1) followed by exposure to open air for 1 h before use [4].

3.3.1 Preparation of Enzymatic Reaction Mixture

(1) Prepare different concentrations of soluble starch concentration in test tubes.
(2) Ensure 10 mL of starch solution in a test tube.
(3) Add 20 alginate beads in each test tube.
(4) Keep the mixtures in an incubator shaker for 10 min at 37°C.
(5) Analyze the sample for the estimation of residual starch.

3.4 Observation

Table 3.1 Concentration of starch after the reaction for 10 min

Initial bulk starch concentration (g/L)	Final bulk starch concentration (g/L)
60	57.979
30	28.046
28	26.062
26	24.065
24	22.065
22	20.088
20	18.097
18	16.106
16	14.115
14	12.141
12	10.172
10	8.217
8	6.319
6	4.546
4	2.926
2	1.470
1	0.728

3.5 Calculated Data

At a high substrate concentration, from Eq. 3.9, we get

$$\text{Slope} = \frac{K_m}{v_{max}}$$

Table 3.2   Calculated data

Initial bulk starch concentration (g/L) (S_b)	Final bulk starch concentration (g/L)	Rate of reaction (g/L min) (v)	$1/S_b$	$1/v$
60	57.979	0.202	0.017	4.95
30	28.046	0.195	0.033	5.12
28	26.062	0.193	0.036	5.16
26	24.065	0.193	0.038	5.17
24	22.065	0.193	0.042	5.17
22	20.088	0.191	0.045	5.232
20	18.097	0.190	0.050	5.256
18	16.106	0.189	0.055	5.28
16	14.115	0.188	0.062	5.304
14	12.141	0.186	0.07	5.38
12	10.172	0.183	0.083	5.47
10	8.217	0.178	0.1	5.61
8	6.319	0.168	0.125	5.952
6	4.546	0.145	0.167	6.88
4	2.926	0.107	0.25	9.312
2	1.470	0.053	0.5	18.88
1	0.728	0.027	1	36.8

$$\text{Intercept} = \frac{1}{v_{\max}}$$

At a high substrate concentration, from Eq. 3.8, we get

$$\text{Slope} = \frac{K_m}{v_{\max}} + \frac{1}{k_a a_m}$$

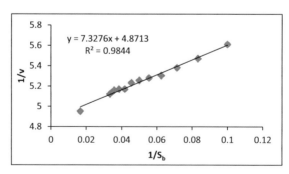

Figure 3.2   Plot of $1/v$ versus $1/S_b$ at a high substrate concentration.

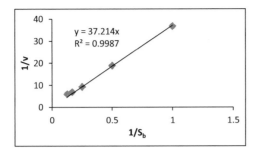

Figure 3.3 Plot of $1/v$ versus $1/S_b$ at low substrate concentrations.

From Fig. 3.2, we get

$$\text{Intercept} = \frac{1}{v_{max}} = 4.8713$$

$$v_{max} = 0.205 \text{ g/L min}$$

$$\text{Slope} = \frac{K_m}{v_{max}} = 7.3276$$

$$K_m = 1.502 \text{ g/L}$$

At a low substrate concentration

$$\text{Slope} = \frac{K_m}{v_{max}} + \frac{1}{k_a a_m} = 37.214$$

$$k_a a_m = 2.00 \text{ h}^{-1}$$

The overall plot of the immobilized enzymatic reaction is shown in Fig. 3.4.

3.6 Discussion

The Lineweaver–Burk plots of the enzymatic reactions using free and immobilized enzyme differ from each other, particularly as high substrate concentration. In the case of an immobilized enzyme, a new parameter such as the rate of diffusion of substrate or product is to be taken into consideration. The effect of diffusion can be monitored by using parameters such as volumetric mass transfer diffusion ($k_a a_m$), effectiveness factor, and Damköhler number. The diffusion problem can be neglected when the effectiveness number

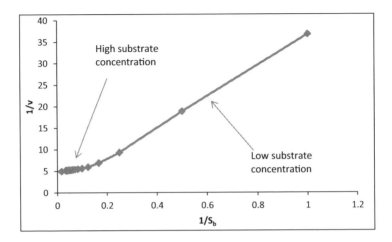

Figure 3.4 Plot of $1/v$ versus $1/S_b$.

approaches 1. In the present experimental study, the second two parameters have not been taken into consideration.

References

1. Das, D. and Das, D., *Biochemical Engineering: An Introductory Textbook*, Jenny Stanford Publishing, Singapore, 2019.
2. Bailey, J. E. and Ollis, D. F., *Biochemical Engineering Fundamentals*, McGraw-Hill Inc., New Delhi, India, 2010.
3. Doran, P. M., *Bioprocess Engineering Principles*, Second Edition, Academic Press, Waltham, USA, 2012.
4. Levenspiel, O., *Chemical Reaction Engineering*, Third Edition, Wiley India, 2010.

Experiment 4

Cell Growth Kinetics in Controlled Fermenter

Objective: To determine cell growth kinetics parameters

4.1 Introduction

The microorganism and the medium play most important roles in the microbial fermentation process. To handle any microorganism, it is necessary to determine the life cycle of the microorganism. Since the microorganisms are mostly active in the log phase, it is necessary to inoculate the seed culture in between the mid-log phase and the late-log phase. Cell growth kinetics parameters are essential to know the growth characteristics of the microorganism.

Prerequisite: Controlled fermenter

4.2 Theory

Growth is the most essential response of microbes to their physio-chemical environment. In a suitable nutrient medium, microbes

Biochemical Engineering: A Laboratory Manual
Debabrata Das and Debayan Das
Copyright © 2021 Jenny Stanford Publishing Pte. Ltd.
ISBN 978-981-4877-36-7 (Hardcover), 978-1-003-11105-4 (eBook)
www.jennystanford.com

extract nutrients from the medium and convert them into biological compounds. As a result of this nutrient utilization, microbial mass increases with time. The material balance of the process can be written as

Substrates + Cells → Extracellular products + More cells

Microbial growth is an example of an auto-catalyzing reaction. The kinetics of cell growth can be determined by using the Monod equation when cells grow on a limiting substrate in an appropriate environment of oxygen, nitrogen source, carbon source, pH, and growth factor (if necessary) as follows:

$$\mu = \frac{\mu_{max} S}{K_S + S} \tag{4.1}$$

where μ is the specific growth rate (h^{-1}), μ_{max} is the maximum specific growth rate (h^{-1}), S is the limiting substrate concentration (g/L), and K_s is the saturation constant specific to the limiting substrate (g/L).

The Monod equation (Eq. 4.1) can be written as

$$\frac{1}{\mu} = \left(\frac{K_S}{\mu_{max}}\right)\frac{1}{s} + \frac{1}{\mu_{max}} \tag{4.2}$$

A plot of $1/\mu$ and $1/s$ gives a straight line with K_s/μ_{max} as slope and $1/\mu_{max}$ as intercept of the line with Y-axis.

When the microbial cells are in the stationary phase, little substrate is available, and endogenous metabolism of the biomass component is used for maintenance energy. Cellular maintenance represents energy expenditures to repair damaged cellular compound, cell motility to adjust osmolality of cell, etc.

This can be mathematically expressed using the Pirt model

$$\left(\frac{ds}{dt}\right)_{overall} = \left(\frac{ds}{dt}\right)_{growth} + \left(\frac{ds}{dt}\right)_{maintenance} \tag{4.3}$$

Maintenance energy is required for cell motility

$$\frac{1}{Y_{x/s}} = \frac{1}{y'_{x/s}} + \frac{m}{\mu} \tag{4.4}$$

where $Y_{x/s}$ is the overall yield coefficient (g cell/g substrate consumed), $y'_{x/s}$ is the true yield coefficient (g cell/g substrate consumed only for growth), m is the maintenance coefficient (time^{-1}), and μ is the specific growth rate of the cell (time^{-1}).

In a batch culture as long as s is adequately large, the cells grow at constant valve of μ, which is always less than μ_{max}.

The log phase growth is given by

$$\left(\frac{dx}{dt}\right) = \mu x \tag{4.5}$$

Integrating

$$\int_{x_0}^{x} \frac{dx}{x} = \int_{0}^{t} \mu dt \Rightarrow \ln x = \ln x_0 + \mu t \tag{4.6}$$

where x is the cell mass concentration at time $t(g/L)$, x_0 is the initial cell mass concentration, and x is the cell mass concentration at time t.

We get a linear curve in the $\ln x$ versus t plot with μ as slope and $\ln x_0$ as intercept.

From Eq. 4.6, we can write doubling time,

$$t_d = \frac{1}{\mu} \int_{x_0}^{2x_0} \frac{dx}{x} = \frac{\ln 2}{\mu} \tag{4.7}$$

Again, minimum doubling time is

$$t_{d,min} = \frac{\ln 2}{\mu_{max}} \tag{4.8}$$

The growth yield coefficient is given by

$$Y_{x/s} = \frac{dS}{dx} = \frac{\Delta S}{\Delta x}$$
$$\Rightarrow \quad Y_{x/s} = \frac{x_2 - x_1}{s_2 - s_1} \tag{4.9}$$

The log phase is a period of balanced growth where the cell growth is more or less uniform. $Y_{x/s}$ remains fairly constant during the log growth phase [1–5].

4.3 Data Table

All data must be presented in a tabular form (Table 4.1).

Table 4.1 Substrate and cell mass concentration at different time intervals

S1 #	Growth time (h)	NTU cells	Concentration of cells, x (g/L)	O.D. for glucose	Concentration of glucose (S) (g/L)	dx/dS ($Y_{x/S}$)

4.3.1 Calculated Data

Plot x and S versus t separately and compute μ for five data points.

Table 4.2 Calculated values of specific growth rate and overall yield coefficients

Data point #	μ	S	$1/\mu$	$1/S$	$1/Y_{x/S}$	x

From the plot of $1/\mu$ vs. $1/S$, one can get K_S/μ_{max} from the slope and $1/\mu_{max}$, from the intercept of y-axis. Similarly, from the plot $1/Y_{x/S}$ vs. $1/\mu$, one can get m from the slope and $Y'_{x/S}$ from the intercept.

The values of dx/dt and dS/dt can be determined by using the differential technique as follows:

$$\frac{dx}{dt} = \frac{x_{n+1} - x_{n-1}}{2\,\Delta t} \tag{4.10}$$

$$\frac{dS}{dt} = \frac{S_{n+1} - S_{n-1}}{2\,\Delta t} \tag{4.11}$$

where n is the sampling number and t is the sampling time interval.

In the discussion of results include:

- The possible effects of contamination of the culture,
- Contamination problems, and
- Your comments on the difference between the K_m of the Michaelis–Menten equation and the K_S of the Monod equation.

Experiment 4A

Cell Growth Kinetics of Bacteria in a Batch Process

Objective: To determine the kinetic parameters for the growth of *Enterobacter cloacae* IIT-BT 08

4A.1 Purpose

To study the cell growth kinetics of bacteria in a batch process and to measure the following kinetic parameters:

- Maximum specific growth rate (μ_{max})
- Saturation constant (K_s)
- True growth yield coefficient ($Y'_{x/S}$)
- Maintenance coefficient (m)

4A.2 Apparatus Required

Fermenter: BIOENGINEERING KLF 2000

Centrifuge: Eppendorf centrifuge 5180R

Vortex: SPHINIX

Spectrophotometer: Nova spec II visible Spectrophotometer

Biochemical Engineering: A Laboratory Manual
Debabrata Das and Debayan Das
Copyright © 2021 Jenny Stanford Publishing Pte. Ltd.
ISBN 978-981-4877-36-7 (Hardcover), 978-1-003-11105-4 (eBook)
www.jennystanford.com

Beaker, conical flask, measuring cylinder, spatula, cotton plug, Eppendorf tube, pipette

4A.3 Medium Preparation

Microorganism: *E. cloacae* IIT-BT 08 (Fig. 4.1)

Type: Facultative anaerobe and rod shape

Growth medium: Nutrient broth production medium
  → MYG (Complex Medium)

M: malt extract; G: glucose; Y: yeast extracts

Total volume of medium to be prepared = 2 L

4A.3.1 Composition of the Medium

Malt extract (1% w/v) = 20 g malt extract in 1.8 L water

Glucose (1% w/v) = 20 g glucose in 1.8 L water

Yeast extract (0.4% w/v) = 8 g in 1.8 L water

Medium volume = 1.8 L

Culture volume = 200 mL

Total working volume = 2 L

4A.3.2 Procedure for Medium Preparation

(1) A conical flask is filled with about 1 L water.
(2) To the conical flask containing water, 20 g of glucose is weighted and added.
(3) Similarly, 20 g malt extract and 8 g of yeast extract are weighed and added to it.
(4) The volume is made up to 1.8 L by adding water.
(5) The prepared medium is auto-calved at 15 psi 121°C for 15 min.
(6) After autoclaving, the medium is allowed to cool.
(7) To make the volume up to 2 L, 200 mL of *E. cloacae* culture grown overnight is added to the medium.

(8) The culture is allowed to grow in the prepared medium incubated in incubator overnight.

4A.3.3 Procedure for the Operation of the Fermenter

(1) The feed port of the Biozenik fermenter (Fig. 4.2) is opened and flamed with spirit lamp to avoid contamination.

(2) The mouth of the conical flask containing culture and medium is also flamed and the reaction mixture is slowly emptied in the fermenting vessel.

(3) The compressor is turned on the control unit of the fermenter and the pH, temperature, impeller speed, rotameter speed values are set.
Speed of impeller: 250 rpm, pH $= 6.7$
Temperature: 30°C

(4) Immediately after turning on the fermenter, 2 mL of sample is collected.
For collecting the sample, the exhaust air filter is closed, and the sample port is opened. Once the pressure in the vessel increases, the sample slowly comes out through the sample port. After taking 2 mL, the sample port is closed, and the exhaust air filter is opened.

(5) After 1 h, sample is collected again by repeating the same process. Around 2–3 mL of the sample in the port is drained as it might have been accumulated the previous time. Then the fresh sample is collected.

(6) The sampling process is done eight times.

(7) The collected samples are centrifuged at 6000 rpm for 15 min.

(8) The supernatant is separated from the pellet and is collected for further test.

4A.4 Determination of Substrate Concentration

4A.4.1 Glucose Estimation by Dinitrosalicylic Acid (DNS)

(1) In different test tubes/Eppendorf tube, 20 μL of each supernatant sample is taken and the volume is made up to 1 mL by adding 980 μL of water.

(2) To each Eppendorf tube, 1 mL of DNA reagents is added.
(3) The mixture is heated for 5–10 min till it develops a red brown color.
(4) To stabilize the color, 1 mL of Rochelle's salt is added (40% sodium potassium tartrate).
(5) The mixture is allowed to cool at cold water bath and the absorbance is recorded with a spectrophotometer at 540 nm.

4A.4.2 Determination of Cell Mass Concentration

(1) The pellet in each Eppendorf tube is washed with 0.85% w/v saline water (0.85 NaCl in 100 mL water).
(2) After adding saline solution, it is vortexed and then centrifuged at 6000 rpm for about 10 min.
(3) The supernatant is drained, and the process is repeated one more time.
(4) After washing the second time, saline water is again added to the pellet and is vortexed.
(5) The absorbance is recorded at 600 nm.

4A.5 Observation

E. cloacae was found to be rod shaped and Gram-negative bacteria.

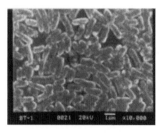

Figure 4.1 SEM photograph of *E. cloacae* (40×).

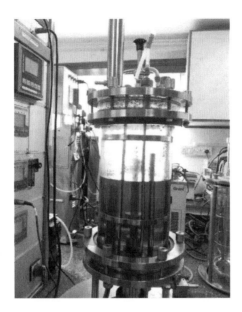

Figure 4.2   Photograph of the controlled fermenter with sterilized medium before the fermentation.

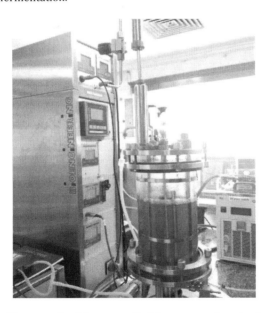

Figure 4.3   Photograph of the controlled fermenter after the fermentation using *E. cloacae.*

Table 4.3 Biomass and glucose concentration at different time

Time (h)	OD at 540 nm	Dilution factor	Glucose (g/L)	OD at 600 nm	Biomass (g/L)
0	0.616	100×	15.4	0.06032	0.13
1	0.6	100×	15	0.079808	0.172
2	0.516	100×	12.9	0.15312	0.33
3	0.392	100×	9.8	0.35728	0.77
4	0.302	100×	7.56	0.638	1.375
5	0.235	100×	5.87	1.0092	2.175
6	0.194	100×	4.86	1.51728	3.27
7	0.173	100×	4.32	1.6936	3.65
8	0.166	100×	4.16	1.75392	3.78

Cell mass concentration (*E. cloacae* IIT-BT 08) and glucose concentration calibration curve under aerobic growth condition depicted in Fig. 4.4 and Fig. 4.5, respectively.

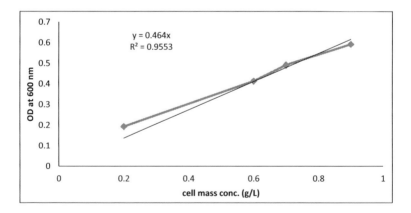

Figure 4.4 Biomass calibration curve of *E. cloacae* IIT-BT 08.

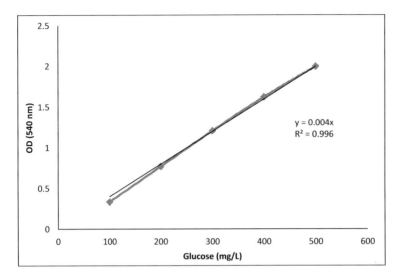

Figure 4.5 Calibration curve of glucose.

4A.6 Calculated Data

Table 4.4 Calculated values of specific growth rate and overall yield coefficient

Time (h)	Biomass (x) (g/L)	Substrate (S) (g/L)	$\dfrac{dx}{dt}$	$\mu = \dfrac{1}{x}\dfrac{dx}{dt}$	$\dfrac{1}{S}$	$\dfrac{1}{\mu}$	$Y_{x/S}$	$\dfrac{1}{Y_{x/S}}$
0	0.13	15.4	—	—	0.065	—	—	—
1	0.17	15.0	0.1	0.58	0.067	1.720	0.100	9.524
2	0.33	12.9	0.299	0.91	0.077	1.104	0.080	12.5
3	0.77	9.8	0.5225	0.68	0.102	1.474	0.114	8.75
4	1.37	7.56	0.7025	0.51	0.132	1.957	0.159	6.297
5	2.17	5.87	0.9475	0.43	0.170	2.295	0.214	4.660
6	3.27	4.86	0.7375	0.22	0.206	4.434	0.298	3.357
7	3.65	4.32	0.255	0.07	0.231	14.313	0.318	3.148
8	3.78	4.16	—	—	0.240	—	0.325	3.079

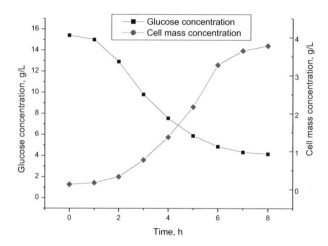

Figure 4.6 Substrate and cell mass concentration profiles.

4A.6.1 Sample Calculation

At time $(t) = 1\,h$

$$x_n = 0.17\,g/L$$

$$X_{n-1} = 0.13\,g/L; X_{n+1} = 0.33\,g/L$$

$$\frac{dx}{dt} = \frac{X_{n+1} - X_{n-1}}{2\Delta t} = \frac{0.33 - 0.13}{2} = 0.1\,g/L\,h$$

$$\mu = \frac{1}{x}\frac{dx}{dt} = \frac{1}{0.17} \times 0.1 = 0.58h^{-1}$$

$$Y_{x/s} = -\left(\frac{x_n - x_{n-1}}{s_n - s_{n-1}}\right) = \frac{0.17 - 0.13}{15.4 - 15.0} = \frac{0.04}{0.04} = 0.1\,g/g$$

From Fig. 4.6, we get Slope $= 8.6881 = \frac{K_s}{\mu_{max}}$ and intercept $=$ $0.7563 = \frac{1}{\mu_{max}}$.

We get

$$\mu_{max} = 1.32\,h^{-1}, K_s = 11.48\,g/L$$

$$t_{d, min} = \frac{\ln 2}{\mu_{max}} = 32.44\,min$$

From Fig. 4.8, the intercept $= \frac{1}{Y'_{x/s(growth)}} = 2.1612, Y'_{x/s(growth)} =$ $0.46\,g/g$.

And the slope $= m = 0.078h^{-1}$.

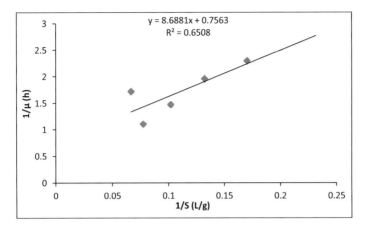

Figure 4.7 Lineweaver–Burk plot to determine the cell growth kinetics constants.

Table 4.5 Values of the cell growth constants

Parameters	Values
$\mu_{max}(\mathrm{h}^{-1})$	1.32
$K_s(\mathrm{g/L})$	11.48
$t_d(\mathrm{min})$	32.44

Table 4.6 Calculated values of maintenance coefficient and true yield coefficient

Parameters	Values
m	$0.078\,\mathrm{h}^{-1}$
$Y'_{x/s}$ (true)	$0.46\,\mathrm{g/g}$

4A.7 Discussion

4A.7.1 Possible Effect of Contamination of the Culture by an Organism with Value of Doubling Time of the Cell, t_d

If the culture gets contaminated by an organism with the same doubling time, then the cell mass doubling time will be the same as that of the uncontaminated culture.

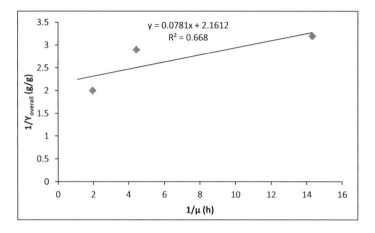

Figure 4.8 Plot of $1/Y_{x/S}$ versus $1/\mu$.

Let $(\frac{dx}{dt})$ be the rate of cell mass growth without contamination.
Now due to contamination

$$\left(\frac{dx}{dt}\right)_{new} = \frac{2dx}{dt}$$

$$\Rightarrow \mu_{new} = \frac{1}{x_{new}}\left(\frac{dx}{dt}\right)_{new} = \frac{1}{2x}\frac{2dx}{dt} = \frac{1}{x}\frac{dx}{dt} = \mu$$

So the specific growth rate remains same.

4A.7.2 Contamination Problems

Bacterial fermentations are prone to several types of contamination.

Bacteriophage contamination may cause the most devastating effect usually resulting in destruction of bacteria culture with subsequent contamination due to sampling or leakage. Failure may be due to extensive foaming and possible chocking of the exhaust filter.

However, bacterial contamination is also common. Sometimes due to mishandling of apparatus and improper lab techniques, new or other bacteria can get introduced. This may lead to reduced yield of product and possible contamination by metabolites of the contaminating bacteria. In some cases, toxins may be produced by contaminants. Cleanup and prevention of these problems remain a considerable challenge.

Due to the relatively low growth rate of yeast and fungi as compared to bacteria, yeast and fungal contamination does not have any effect on bacterial fermentation.

4A.7.3 Difference between K_m and K_s

K_m is the Michaelis–Menten constant, which shows the concentration of the substrate with the reaction velocity equal to half of the maximal velocity for the reaction. K_m is also a measure of substrates affinity. Low K_m indicates large building affinity.

K_s is the Monod constant, which is numerically equal to the substrate concentration when the specific growth rate is exactly half the maximum specific growth rate. Low value of K_s and high value of μ_{max} result in higher cell growth.

4A.8 Conclusion

From the graph we can conclude that cell mass concentration increases with time, while substrate (glucose) concentration decreases with time. However, there were mild fluctuations in the data obtained. This may be due to several reasons. The sample might have been contaminated by some slow-growing microbe whose presence could not be traced at the beginning. Some of microbes might have been washed away when washing the pellet with saline water. Another glucose estimation method may be required for crosschecking the glucose concentration of the samples, such as the glucose oxidase method.

References

1. Das, D. and Das, D., *Biochemical Engineering: An Introductory Textbook*, Jenny Stanford Publishing, Singapore, 2019.
2. Bailey, J. E. and Ollis, D. F., *Biochemical Engineering Fundamentals*, McGraw-Hill Inc., New Delhi, India, 2010.

3. Doran, P. M. *Bioprocess Engineering Principles*, Second Edition, Academic Press, Waltham, USA, 2012.

4. Shuler, M. L. and Kargi, F. *Bioprocess Engineering: Basic Concepts*, Second Edition, Prentice-Hall Inc., New Delhi, India, 2002.

5. Nath, K. and Das, D. Modeling and optimization of fermentative hydrogen production, *Bioresource Technology*, **102**: 8569–8581, 2011.

Experiment 4B

Cell Growth Kinetics of Yeast in a Batch Process

Objective: To determine the kinetic parameters for the growth of *Saccharomyces cerevisiae*

4B.1 Purpose

To determine the following cell growth kinetics of yeast in a batch system and to measure

- Maximum specification growth (μ_{max})
- Saturation constant (K_s)
- Growth yield coefficient ($Y_{x/s}$)
- Maintenance coefficient (m)

4B.2 Background Statement

Microbe: *Saccharomyces cerevisiae*

Species: Yeast

Biochemical Engineering: A Laboratory Manual
Debabrata Das and Debayan Das
Copyright © 2021 Jenny Stanford Publishing Pte. Ltd.
ISBN 978-981-4877-36-7 (Hardcover), 978-1-003-11105-4 (eBook)
www.jennystanford.com

Type: Eukaryotic organism (aerobic condition)

Ecology: Found primarily on ripe fruits

Optimum temperature: 30–35°C

Life cycle: Haploid cells undergo a simple life cycle of mitosis and growth (budding)

Diploid cells can either undergo mitosis or sporulation by entering meiosis and producing four haploid spores.

Doubling time: (99 ± 1) min

Nutritional requirements: Can grow aerobically on glucose, maltose and trehalose, ammonia, urea, amino acids, peptides, phosphorous, and sulfur; can be assimilated as SO_4^{2-} or as organic sulfur; some metals such as magnesium, iron, calcium, and zinc are also required for good growth of the yeast.

Most strains also require biotin and pantothenate for cell growth.

Cell growth: Growth in yeast is synchronized with the growth of the bud, which reaches the size of the mature cell by the time. It separates from the parent cell. In well-nourished, rapidly growing yeast cells, all the cells can be seen to have buds, since bud formation occupies the whole cell cycle (Fig. 4.9).

4B.3 Apparatus Required

Fermenter: New Brunswick Bio flow 110 (in vitro autoclave fermenter)

Centrifuge: Eppendorf centrifuge 5180 R

Vortex: SPHINIX

Spectrophotometer: Nova spec II visible spectrophotometer shaking incubator

Beaker, conical flask, measuring cylinder, weight balance, spatula, Eppendorf, pipette, test tubes, Bunsen burner.

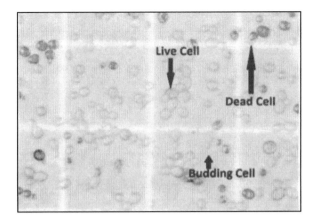

Figure 4.9 Morphology of yeast cell (*S. cerevisiae*) at 40× magnification (dye is methylene blue).

4B.4 Medium Preparation

Type: Complex medium

Ingredients: Yeast extract (4 g/L), peptone (10 g/L), dextrose (10 g/L)

Total working volume = 2 L

(1) A conical flask is filled with 1 L water.
(2) To the conical flask containing water, 20 g dextrose is weighed and added.
(3) Similarly, 20 g of peptone and 8 g of yeast extract are weighed and added to the flask.
(4) The volume is made up to 1.8 L by adding water.
(5) The mouth of the conical flask is sealed with cotton plug.
(6) The prepared medium is autoclaved at 15 psi, 121°C for 15 min.
(7) After autoclaving, the medium is allowed to cool.

4B.5 Culture Preparation

(1) The yeast culture is stored at 4°C. It is grown on an agar plate.

(2) One loop of culture is taken and added to YPD medium in laminar air flow to avoid any contamination.

(3) The culture and medium are incubated at 30°C in an incubator shaker for about 10 h.

The inoculum is now ready to use.

(1) To make the total volume up to 2 L, 200 mL of the grown culture is added to 1.8 L of YPD medium.

(2) The culture and medium are kept at 30°C for about 6–8 h in the incubator shaker and is then transferred to the fermenter.

This procedure is followed to skip the lag phase in the final culture and medium. Before the addition of the mixture to the fermenter, all cells attain the mid-log phase.

4B.5.1 Procedure

(1) The feed portion of the fermenter is opened and flamed to avoid contamination.

(2) The mouth of the conical flask containing culture and medium is also flamed, and the reaction mixture is slowly emptied in the fermenting vessel with flaming.

(3) The air pump is switched on. The motor and the controlling unit of the fermenter are turned on.

(4) The temperature is maintained at 30°C for optimum growth sampling.

(5) Immediately after turning on the fermenter, 2 mL of sample is collected. For collecting the sample, (a) the air outlet is closed and (b) the sample port is opened due to increase in pressure; the sample slowly rises and comes out of the sample port. After collecting 2 mL of the sample, the sample port is closed and the aeration outlet is opened.

(6) After 1 h, a sample is again collected by repeating the same procedure. About 2–3 mL of the sample coming out of the port is initially drained out as it might have been accumulated during the previous sampling. The fresh sample is then collected.

(7) The sampling process is done about eight times.
(8) The samples collected are centrifuged at above 6000 rpm for 15 min.
(9) The supernatant is separated from the pellet and is collected in test tubes for further test.

4B.5.2 Cell Mass Concentration Estimation

(1) To 100 mL of water, 0.85 g of NaCl is added to make 0.85% w/v saline water for washing the cells off any salts, minerals, or trace of medium.
(2) Saline water is added to each Eppendorf tube containing the pellet and is vortexed to mix the cells in saline water.
(3) It is then centrifuged at 6000 rpm for 10 min. The supernatant is drained off.
(4) The process is repeated one more time.
(5) After the process of washing for the second time, saline water is again added to the pellet and is vortexed.
(6) The absorbance is recorded at 600 nm.

4B.5.3 Glucose Estimation

Estimation of reducing sugar present in the fermentation sample by the dinitrosalicylic acid (DNS) method.

(1) From each Eppendorf tube, 20 μL of supernatant is taken and added to a clean, dry test tube and is diluted 50 times by adding 980 μL of water and the volume is made up to 1 mL.
(2) To each Eppendorf tube, 1 mL of DNS reagent is added.
(3) The mixture is heated for 5–10 min till it develops an orange-red color.
(4) To stabilize the color, 1 mL of Rochelle's salt is added (40% w/v sodium potassium tartrate).
(5) The mixture is allowed to cool, and absorbance is recorded at 540 nm.

4B.6 Observation

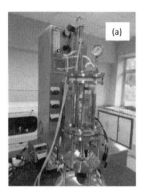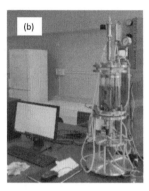

Figure 4.10 Controlled fermenter (a) without medium and (b) with the sterilized medium before the fermentation.

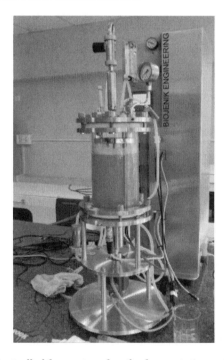

Figure 4.11 Controlled fermenter after the fermentation using *S. cerevisiae*.

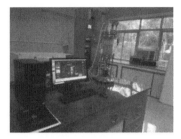

Figure 4.12 Biozenik fermenter with the computer control system (SOPs are in the Appendices).

Table 4.7 Change in cell mass and glucose concentration with respect to time

Time (h)	OD at 540 nm	Dilution factor	Glucose (g/L)	OD at 600 nm	Biomass (g/L)
0	0.508	100×	12.7	0.045	0.1
1	0.502	100×	12.55	0.090	0.2
2	0.475	100×	11.87	0.226	0.5
3	0.432	100×	10.8	0.635	1.4
4	0.336	100×	8.4	0.951	2.1
5	0.216	100×	5.4	1.178	2.6
6	0.107	100×	2.67	1.50	3.31
7	0.046	100×	1.15	1.658	3.66
8	0.022	100×	0.55	1.768	3.9
9	0.02	100×	0.5	1.813	4.0
10	0.016	100×	0.4	1.903	4.2

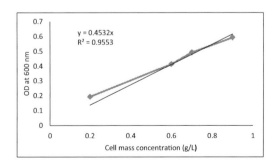

Figure 4.13 Calibration curve for the cell mass concentration.

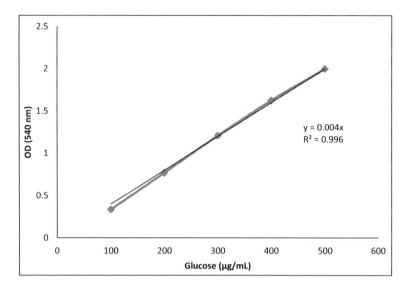

Figure 4.14   Calibration curve of standard glucose solution.

4B.7 Calculated Data

Table 4.8   Calculated data for the determination of μ_{max} and K_S

Time (h)	Biomass (x) (g/L)	Substrate (S) (g/L)	$\dfrac{dx}{dt}$	$\mu = \dfrac{1}{x}\dfrac{dx}{dt}$	$\dfrac{1}{S}$	$\dfrac{1}{\mu}$	$Y_{x/S(overall)}$	$\dfrac{1}{Y_{x/S(overall)}}$
0	0.1	12.7	—	—	—	—	—	—
1	0.2	12.55	0.2	1	0.08	1	0.67	1.5
2	0.5	11.87	0.6	0.12	0.08	0.83	0.48	2.07
3	1.4	10.8	0.8	0.57	0.09	1.75	0.68	1.46
4	2.1	8.4	0.7	0.33	0.12	3	0.46	2.15
5	2.8	5.4	0.60	0.22	0.18	4.63	0.37	2.70
6	3.31	2.67	0.43	0.13	0.37	7.70	0.32	3.12
7	3.66	1.15	0.29	0.08	0.87	12.41	0.31	3.24
8	3.9	0.55	0.17	0.04	1.82	22.94	0.31	3.20
9	4	0.5	0.15	0.04	2.0	26.67	0.32	3.13
10	4.2	0.4	—	—	2.5	—	—	—

4B.7.1 Sample Calculation

At time $= 2$ h

$$x_n = 0.5\,\text{g/L},\ x_{n-1} = 0.2\,\text{g/L},\ x_{n+1} = 1.4\,\text{g/L}$$

$$S_n = 11.87\text{g/L},\ S_{n-1} = 12.55\,\text{g/L},\ S_{n+1} = 10.8\,\text{g/L}$$

$$\frac{dx}{dt} = \frac{X_{n+1} - X_{n-1}}{2\Delta t} = \frac{1.4 - 0.2}{2} = 0.6\,\text{g/L h}$$

$$\mu = \frac{1}{x_n}\frac{dx}{dt} = \frac{1}{0.5} \times 0.6 = 0.12\,\text{h}^{-1}$$

$$Y_{x/s} = \frac{x_t - x_0}{S_0 - S_t} = \frac{0.5 - 0.1}{12.7 - 11.87} = 0.48$$

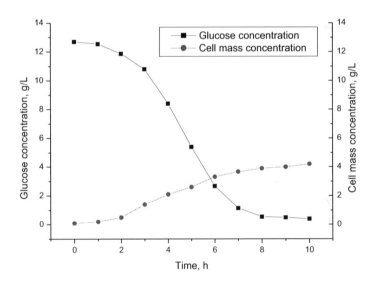

Figure 4.15   Substrate and cell mass concentration profiles.

From Eq. 4.2,

$$\frac{1}{\mu} = \left(\frac{K_s}{\mu_{\max}}\right)\frac{1}{s} + \frac{1}{\mu_{\max}}$$

From Fig. 4.16, the intercept is $\frac{1}{\mu_{\max}} = 2.5064$.

$$\mu_{\max} = 0.399\,\text{h}^{-1}$$

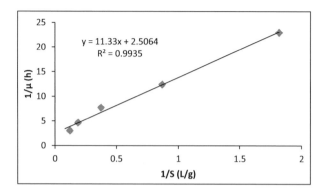

Figure 4.16 Plot of $1/\mu$ versus $1/S$.

$$t_{d,min} = \frac{\ln 2}{\mu_{max}} = 104 \text{ min}$$

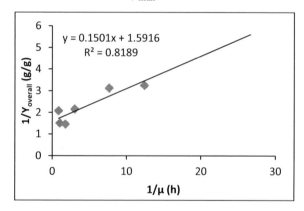

Figure 4.17 Plot of $1/Y_{x/s}$ versus $1/\mu$.

Again, from the slope, $\frac{K_S}{\mu_{max}} = 11.33$

$$K_s = 4.52 \text{g/L}$$

$$t_{d,min} = \frac{\ln 2}{\mu_{max}} = 104 \text{ min}$$

The Pirt equation (Eq. 4.4) is

$$\frac{1}{Y_{x/s}} = \frac{1}{y'_{x/s}} + \frac{m}{\mu}$$

From Fig. 4.17, the intercept is $\frac{1}{y'_{x/s}} = 1.5916$.

$$Y'_{x/s \text{ (growth)}} = 0.63 \text{ g/g}$$

$$m = 0.15 \text{ h}^{-1}$$

Results are tabulated in Table 4.9 [1–3].

Table 4.9 Kinetic constants of *S. cerevisiae*

Kinetic parameters	Values
μ_{max}	0.399 h^{-1}
K_s	4.52 g/L
t_d	104 min
$Y'_{x/s(g)}$	0.63
m	0.15 h^{-1}

4B.8 Discussion

4B.8.1 Contamination Problems

Yeast fermentation is prone to bacterial contamination. Bacteria are usually fast growing in comparison to slow-growing yeast population. Bacteria tend to utilize the nutrients meant for yeast. Bacteria can grow in the optimal condition meant for yeast growth. Due to the consumption of nutrients by the bacterial population, yeasts face lack of nutrients in a batch culture and yeast growth is hampered. The turbidity is mostly due to bacterial growth.

However, a certain scientific study indicates that bacteriophages may be regarded as an antimicrobial agent or in conjunction with antibiotics in the yeast fermentation process. Implementation of bacteriophages with other common contamination abatement/prevention methods can further increase the efficacy of the yeast fermentation process.

4B.8.2 Issue of Alcoholic Fermentation

In *S. cerevisiae*, high sugar concentration and high specific growth rate can trigger alcoholic fermentation even under fully aerobic conditions. Alcoholic fermentation during industrial production of Baker's yeast is highly undesirable as it reduces the biomass yield.

Higher biomass productivity is possible in the fed batch process for the use of maximum amount of substrate. In the early stage of the process, the maximum feasible growth rate is dictated by the threshold-specific growth rate at which respirofermentive metabolism sets in. In later stages, the specific growth is decreased to avoid problems with limited oxygen transfer and/or cooling capacity of bioreactors.

The chemostat cultivation system allows the manipulation of the growth rate while keeping other important growth factors constant. Recent studies have portrayed the fact that differences in fermentative capacity between a laboratory strain of *S. cerevisiae* and an industrial strain become apparent only in glucose-limited chemostat culture but not in batch cultures. High concentration of sugar in the batch process may lead to ethanol formation.

Doubling time obtained $= 73$ min

At pH $= 6.5$, temperature $= 30°C$.

Carbon source: Glucose

Theoretical value $= 100$ min (physicochemical parameter not mentioned)

The growth of any microbial cell is highly dependent on the physicochemical parameters. The nutritional state and optimum conditions in which yeast cells are grown in lab may have been different from the ones in the literature. This could be a possible reason for different values. Moreover, the cells of mid-log phase are to be considered an inoculum.

4B.9 Conclusion

From the biomass profile and substrate degradation profile, we can conclude that the biomass increases with time and substrate concentration decreases with time. Substrate concentration decreases with time almost as expected. The doubling time reported for yeast is about 100 min, which is closer to our experimental result. Other kinetic constants are closer to those reported in the literature. So it can be concluded that there is little chance of contamination during the experimental studies.

References

1. Das, D. and Das, D., *Biochemical Engineering: An Introductory Textbook*, Jenny Stanford Publishing, Singapore, 2019.
2. Bailey, J. E. and Ollis, D. F., *Biochemical Engineering Fundamentals*, McGraw-Hill Inc., New Delhi, India, 2010.
3. Doran, P. M., *Bioprocess Engineering Principles*, Second Edition, Academic Press, Waltham, USA, 2012.

Experiment 4C

Cell Growth Kinetics of Microalgae in a Batch Process

Objective: To determine the kinetic parameters for the growth of *Chlorella* sp. MJ 11/11

4C.1 Purpose

To determine the cell growth kinetics of microalgae in a batch system and to measure

- Maximum specific growth rate (μ_{max})
- Saturation constant (K_s)
- Growth yield coefficient ($Y_{x/s}$)
- Maintenance coefficient (m)

4C.2 Background Statement

Microbe: *Chlorella* sp. MJ 11/11

Domain: Eukaryotic

Biochemical Engineering: A Laboratory Manual
Debabrata Das and Debayan Das
Copyright © 2021 Jenny Stanford Publishing Pte. Ltd.
ISBN 978-981-4877-36-7 (Hardcover), 978-1-003-11105-4 (eBook)
www.jennystanford.com

Kingdom: Plantae—algae

Shape: Spherical

Size: 2–10 μm in diameter

Chlorella is an example of microalgae or microphytes that are unicellular species and exist either individually or in chains or groups. Unlike higher plants, microalgae do not have roots, stems, or leaves.

4C.2.1 Modes of Growth

- Autotrophic in the presence of inorganic carbon and light
- Heterotrophic in the presence of organic carbon and absence of light
- Mixotrophic in the presence of organic and inorganic carbon and light

4C.2.2 Cultivation Methods

4C.2.2.1 Open ponds

Raceway-type ponds and lakes are open to the elements. But they are highly vulnerable to contamination. They are cheaper to construct and can exploit unusual conditions that suit specific algae.

4C.2.2.2 Photobioreactor

A photobioreactor is a bioreactor that incorporates a light source. It is a closed system. Since the system is closed, the growing microbe (algae) must be provided with all nutrients, including CO_2.

4C.2.3 Light Intensity

Photochemical reaction in photosynthesis depends on the number of photons incident on the surface and the irradiance as the number of quanta (photons) reaching a unit surface in time. Photosynthetic photon flux density is measured as (μ mol of quanta/m^2s)

$$1 \, \mu \, \text{mol} = 6.023 \times 10^{17} \, \text{photons}$$

4C.3 Theory

When microbial cells are grown in a suitable nutrient medium, they grow by extracting nutrient from the medium and simultaneously convert them into biological compounds. As a result, the substrate concentration decreases with increase in cell biomass.

4C.3.1 Growth-Limiting Substrate

If a medium consists of n compounds, $(n - 1)$ components are fixed and the changes in specific growth rate are observed for the change in concentration of that particular substrate.

If μ initially increases with the substrate concentration but at a particular substrate concentration μ attains its maximum value and any further increase in substrate concentration does not alter the value of specific growth rate, such a substrate is called growth-limiting substrate (Fig. 4.18). A growth-limiting substrate may be a carbon source or nitrogen source or vitamins or minerals present in the medium.

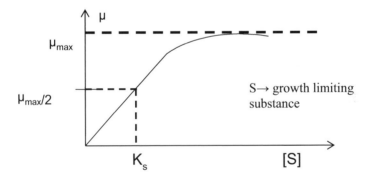

Figure 4.18 Growth cycle of a microbial cell.

When cells are grown in growth-limiting substrate medium, their growth kinetics can be determined experimentally by determining the growth kinetics parameters. The Monod equation for cell growth kinetics and the Pirt equation for the maintenance of the cells have already been discussed [1–3].

4C.4 Process Requirement

- Fermenter: Eppendorf DASGIP Photobioreactor
- Gas chromatography: AutoSystem XL, PerkinElmer, USA
- Quanta meter: LI –COR Bioscience, Sensor model LI-250A
- Column: Elite FFAP
- Spectrophotometer: Amersham Pharmacia Biotech

4C.4.1 Medium

Type: Defined/synthetic medium
   TAP medium: Tris acetate phosphate medium (2.5 L) [6]

- TAP salt stock solution = 12.5 mL/L (v/v) (31.25 mL in 2.5 L)
- Phosphate stock solution = 0.375 mL/L (v/v) (0.94 mL in 2.5 L)
- Hunter trace metals = 1 mL/L (v/v) (2.5 mL in 2.5 L)
- Vitamin stock solution = 1 mL/L (v/v) (2.5 mL in 2.5 L)
- Glacial acetic acid = 1 mL/L (v/v) (2.5 mL in 2.5 L)
- Tris base = 2.42 g/L (6.05 g in 2.5 L)
  (buffer to maintain pH)
- Water is added to make up the remaining volume to 2.5 L.

4C.5 Procedure

4C.5.1 Culture Preparation

(1) For inoculation, a Petri plate with a single-cell colony is taken.
(2) Active organisms are needed. Microorganism is subculture to get the active culture.
(3) When the culture attains the mid-log phase, it is taken in a suspension culture.
(4) The culture is then added to the reaction at 25°C.
   Light intensity = 137.11 μ mol/m^{2}s
   Initial pH of medium = 7.2

Since *Chlorella* is a slow-growing microbe, sample is collected every 12 h.

4C.5.2 Sample Collection Procedure

(1) The exhaust air filter is closed.
(2) The sample port is opened.
(3) Due to increase in pressure in the reactor, the sample slowly comes out through the sample port.
(4) After taking 2 mL of sample, the sample port is closed, and the exhaust air filter is opened.
(5) After 12 h, sample is again collected by repeating the same process. About 2–3 mL of sample in the port is drained as it might have been accumulated the pervious time. Then a fresh sample is collected.
(6) The samples collected are centrifuged at 6000 rpm for 15 min.
(7) The supernatant is separated from the pellet and is collected for further test.
(8) Two samples are collected at a particular time: One set is used for measuring the chlorophyll content, and other set is used for measuring the dry cell weight and substrate concentration.

4C.5.3 Estimation of Chlorophyll Content

(1) To the cell pellet obtained, 1 mL of 95% methanol is added, and it is then stored overnight.
(2) The suspension is then centrifuged as the absorbance of the supernatant is taken at 650 nm and 665 nm against 95% methanol as blank.
(3) The concentration of chlorophyll is estimated using the formula.

4C.5.4 Dry Cell Weight Estimation

(1) Prior to collecting sample at a particular time, the weight of the empty Eppendorf tube is measured.

(2) After all samples are collected, they are centrifuged at 6000 rpm for 15 min for pelleting down the cell mass.
(3) The supernatant is then separated from the pellet.
(4) Distilled water is then added to the pellet to wash off any traces of salt, minerals, or medium present in the pellet. The water is then discarded.
(5) Distilled water is again added, and the mixture is centrifuged at 6000 rpm for 10 min. The mixture is left overnight for drying in the oven at 60°C.
(6) The Eppendorf tube containing the pellets is weighed.
(7) The difference in the weights of the pellet-containing Eppendorf tube and the empty Eppendorf tube is recorded as the dry cell weight.

4C.5.5 Analyzing Substrate Consumption by Gas Chromatography Flame Ionization Detection

The concentration of acetic acid in the supernatant is determined using a gas chromatography equipment with a flame ionization detector (FID) and capillary column (elite – FFAP) coated with 10% PEG-20M and 2% H_3PO_4 (80/100 mesh).

(1) The temperatures of the injection port, oven, detector, and program are set to 220°C, 240°C, 240°C, and 130–175°C, respectively.
(2) Nitrogen is used as the carrier gas at a flow rate of 20 mL/min. The mixture of hydrogen and air at the flow rate of 30 mL/min is used for flame generation.

Chromatographic data are present as a graph of detector response against retention time, called a chromatogram. It provides a spectrum of peak for a sample representing the analyte present in the sample. The area under a peak is proportional to the amount of analyte, i.e., substrate present at a particular time.

4C.6 Observation

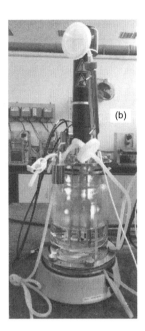
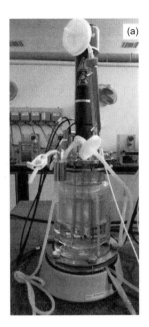

Figure 4.19   Controlled photobioreactor: (a) without light and (b) with LED light before the fermentation.

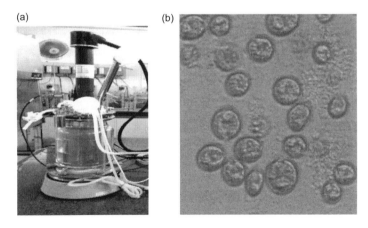

Figure 4.20   (a) Controlled photobioreactor after the fermentation using *Chlorella* sp. and (b) morphology of *Chlorella* sp. under the microscope.

Table 4.10 Experimental data with respect to time

Time (h)	Weight of empty Eppendorf tube (g)	Weight of Eppendorf tube with dry cell mass (g)	Biomass concentration (x) (g/L)	Acetate concentration (S) (mg/L)	Chlorophyll content (mg/L)
0	1.2	1.21	0.03	2000	0.0045
12	1.20	1.20	0.05	1936	0.0113
24	1.21	1.21	0.16	1785	0.0148
36	1.21	1.21	0.38	1534	0.0158
48	1.20	1.20	0.65	1130	0.0162
60	1.21	1.21	0.91	814	0.0163
72	1.22	1.22	1.22	480	0.178
84	1.20	1.20	1.53	255	0.0193
96	1.21	1.21	1.86	105	0.0199
108	1.21	1.22	2.1	90	0.0208
120	1.21	1.22	2.25	74	0.0210
132	1.21	1.21	2.3	55	0.0210
144	1.21	1.22	2.3	54	0.0210

Table 4.11 Experimental and calculated data

Time (h)	Biomass (x) (g/L)	Acetate (S) (mg/L)	S (g/L)	$\dfrac{dx}{dt}$	$\mu = \dfrac{1}{x}\dfrac{dx}{dt}$	$\dfrac{1}{S}$	$\dfrac{1}{\mu}$	$Y'_{x/S}$	$\dfrac{1}{Y'_{x/S}}$
0	0.03	2000	2	—	—	0.5	—	—	—
12	0.05	1936	1.936	0.005	0.1185	0.516	8.44	0.29	3.48
24	0.16	1785	1.785	0.014	0.0868	0.560	11.51	0.61	1.63
36	0.38	1534	1.534	0.020	0.0537	0.652	18.61	0.75	1.32
48	0.65	1130	1.13	0.022	0.0341	0.885	29.32	0.71	1.40
60	0.91	814	0.814	0.024	0.0260	1.228	35.4	0.74	1.34
72	1.22	480	0.48	0.026	0.0211	2.083	47.38	0.78	1.27
84	1.53	255	0.255	0.027	0.0174	3.921	57.37	0.86	1.16
96	1.86	105	0.105	0.024	0.0128	9.524	78.31	0.97	1.03
108	2.1	90	0.09	0.016	0.0077	11.11	129.23	1.08	0.92
120	2.25	74	0.074	0.008	0.0037	13.51	270	1.15	0.87
132	2.3	55	0.055	0.002	0.0009	18.18	1104	1.17	0.86
144	2.3	54	0.054	—	—	18.52	—	1.17	0.86

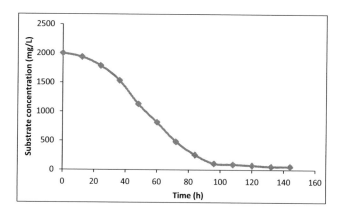

Figure 4.21   Substrate (acetate) concentration profile.

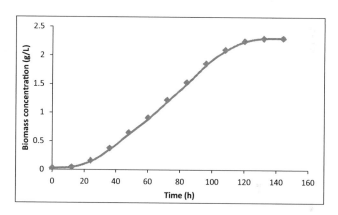

Figure 4.22   Cell mass concentration profile.

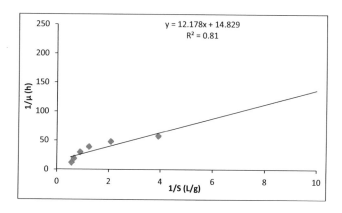

Figure 4.23   Plot of $1/\mu$ versus $1/S$.

From Fig. 4.23, the intercept is $\frac{1}{\mu_{max}} = 14.829$.

$$\mu_{max} = 0.067\,h^{-1}$$

The slope is $\frac{K_S}{\mu_{max}} = 12.178$.

$$K_S = 0.82\,g/L$$

$$t_{d,\,min} = \frac{\ln 2}{\mu_{max}} = 10.34\,h$$

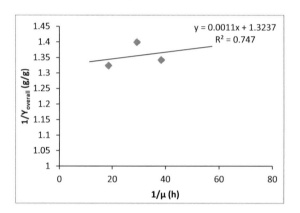

Figure 4.24 Plot of $1/Y_{x/S}$ versus $1/\mu$.

From Fig. 4.24, the intercept is $\frac{1}{Y'_{x/s\,(growth)}} = 1.3237$.

$$Y'_{x/s\,(growth)} = 0.755\,g/g$$

From Fig. 4.24, the intercept is $\frac{1}{Y'_{x/s\,(growth)}} = 1.3609$.

$$m = 0.0011h^{-1}$$

4C.6.1 Sample Calculation

At time $= 24\,h$

Biomass concentration, $x = 0.16\,g/L$

$$X_{n-1} = 0.05\,g/L;\ X_{n+1} = 0.38\,g/L$$

$$\frac{dx}{dt} = \frac{X_{n+1} - X_{n-1}}{2\Delta t} = \frac{0.38 - 0.05}{24} = 0.014\,g/L\,h$$

$$\mu = \frac{1}{x}\frac{dx}{dt} = \frac{0.014}{0.16} = 0.0868\,h^{-1}$$

$$Y_{x/s} = \frac{x_t - x_0}{s_0 - s_t} = \frac{(0.16 - 0.03)}{(2 - 1.785)} = 0.61$$

4C.7 Discussion

In the experiment, the algae are grown in the mixotrophic mode. The medium is provided with an organic carbon source, i.e., acetate, and the growth is carried out in a photobioreactor, which ensured the presence of sufficient amount of light to allow the autotrophic mode of nutrition by photosynthesis. When the organic carbon source is depleted in the medium, the algae shift from the heterotrophic mode of nutrition to autotrophic.

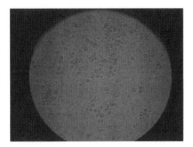

Figure 4.25   Photomicrograph of *Chlorella* sp. MJ 11/11 at 100×.

The culture is prone to contamination by other algal species. They compete with *Chlorella* for nutrients provided in the medium. This hampers their growth by heterotrophic mode of nutrition, and the desired results for substrate consumption are not obtained.

If the culture (algae) gets contaminated by a bacteria culture, it hampers the growth of algae by the heterotrophic mode of nutrition and the desired results for substrate consumption are not obtained. Alga is a slow-growing organism with a doubling time of about 8–10 h, and the doubling time of bacterial culture is about 20–30 min. Since bacteria are fast growing, they consume most of the nutrients present in the medium and decrease the amount of nutrients required for the algae. The bacterial population will also share a major portion in the measured dry cell weight.

Among the environmental factors affecting the growth rate of unicellular algae, light intensity is an important parameter. In many laboratory culture used for physiological research, the light intensity is too low to permit logarithmic growth. High light intensity, temperature, CO_2 level and nutrient supply may influence the growth of microalgae.

Chlorella contains lipids, pigments, carbohydrates, proteins (single-cell proteins), some vitamins such as vitamins A, B2, and B3 and metals such as Fe, Mg, and Zn. In addition, *Chlorella* also contains a good quantity of vitamins B1 and B6 and phosphorous. *Chlorella* is one of the most nutrient-based food. *Chlorella*'s high levels of chlorophyll have been proved to protect the body against UV radiation treatments (chemotherapy) while removing radioactive particles from the body. It helps to regulate hormones helping with metabolism, improving circulation, and promoting higher levels of energy [4–6].

4C.8 Conclusion

Growth characteristics of *Chlorella* sp. is remarkably close to the data reported in the literature. It has been observed from the previous three experimental studies that the doubling time of the organism follows the following trend:

Doubling time bacteria (32.4 min) < Doubling time of yeast (104 min) < Doubling time of microalgae (10.34 h)

A similar trend has also been reported in the literature.

References

1. Das, D. and Das, D., *Biochemical Engineering: An Introductory Textbook*, Jenny Stanford Publishing, Singapore, 2019.
2. Bailey, J. E. and Ollis, D. F., *Biochemical Engineering Fundamentals*, McGraw-Hill Inc., New Delhi, India, 2010.
3. Doran, P. M., *Bioprocess Engineering Principles*, Second Edition, Academic Press, Waltham, USA, 2012.
4. Kumar, K. and Das, D., Growth characteristics of *Chlorella sorokiniana* in airlift and bubble column photobioreactors, *Bioresource Technology*, **116**: 307–313, 2012.

5. Kumar, K., Nag Dasgupta, C., and Das, D., Cell growth kinetics of *Chlorella sorokiniana* and nutritional values of its biomass, *Bioresource Technology*, **167**: 358–366, 2014.

6. Das, D., *Algal Biorefinery: An Integrated Approach*, Capital Publishing Company Ltd Springer, Switzerland, 2015.

Experiment 5

Determination of Volumetric Mass Transfer Coefficient

Objective: To find out the volumetric oxygen transfer coefficient (k_La) of a fermentation process using *Saccharomyces cerevisiae*

5.1 Purpose

To determine the volumetric oxygen transfer coefficient (k_La) of a fermentation process by the dynamic gassing out method using yeast cells.

5.2 Microorganism

Microbe: *Saccharomyces cerevisiae*

Species: Yeast

Kingdom: Fungi

Temperature: $30–35°C$

Fermenter

Biochemical Engineering: A Laboratory Manual
Debabrata Das and Debayan Das
Copyright © 2021 Jenny Stanford Publishing Pte. Ltd.
ISBN 978-981-4877-36-7 (Hardcover), 978-1-003-11105-4 (eBook)
www.jennystanford.com

Nutritional requirements: Can grow aerobically on glucose, maltose, trehalose, ammonia, urea, amino acids, peptides, phosphorous, some metals such as Mg, Fe, Ca, and Zn, and vitamins such as biotin, inositol, and panthenol.

5.3 Theory

When air is sparged through a fermentation medium, a fraction of it remains in the broth as dissolved oxygen (DO), a certain amount is utilized by the cell for its growth, and the rest comes out of the fermenter.

Sparging is basically done to maintain DO concentration in the fermenter to facilitate aerobic growth of the cells.

$$\text{Rate of oxygen transferred} = k_L a \left(C^* - C_L \right) \tag{5.1}$$

where C^* is the saturated dissolved oxygen concentration (mg/L), C_L is the dissolved oxygen concentration of the fermentation broth at any time t (mg/L), and $k_L a$ is the volumetric mass transfer coefficient (time^{-1}) [1–4].

$$\text{Rate of oxygen uptake/consumed by the cell} = Q_{O_2} x \tag{5.2}$$

where Q_{O_2} is the specific oxygen (O_2) uptake rate of cell mass (time^{-1}), x is the cell mass concentration (mg/L).

$$\text{Rate of oxygen dissolution} = \left(\begin{array}{c} \text{Rate of } O_2 \\ \text{transferred} \end{array} \right) - \left(\begin{array}{c} \text{Rate of } O_2 \\ \text{consumed} \\ \text{by cells} \end{array} \right) \tag{5.3}$$

$$\Rightarrow \frac{dC_L}{dt} = k_L a \left(C^* - C_L \right) - Q_{O_2} x \tag{5.4}$$

Equation 5.4 can be written as

$$\left(C^* - C_L \right) = \frac{1}{k_L a} \left(\frac{dC_L}{dt} + Q_{O_2} x \right)$$

$$C_L = C^* - \frac{1}{k_L a} \left(\frac{dC_L}{dt} + Q_{O_2} x \right) \tag{5.5}$$

Before performing the experiment, DO probe calibration is done. It is a two-point calibration.

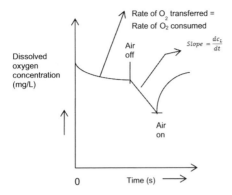

Figure 5.1   DO profile in the fermentation broth.

For 0 %: Fermenter is sparged with N_2. N_2 replaces DO. Once DO is stable, it is set to zero.

For 100%: The fermenter is sparged with air (as pure O_2 is toxic). Once the control unit shows a stable value of DO, it is set to 100%. The saturated DO concentration is 9 mg/L.

The critical DO concentration is 0.2 mg/L. Above the critical level, the O_2 concentration no longer limits the growth, i.e., the specific growth is independent of the DO of the medium. For optimum growth, it is important to maintain this condition. DO levels above the critical value are maintained by sparging the bioreactor with air. The mass transfer rate of oxygen to the liquid broth must equal or exceed the rate at which the growing cells take up that oxygen. During cell culture, O_2 is transferred from gas to liquid so that it can ultimately be absorbed into a cell and consumed. The oxygen transfer rate (OTR) is strongly influenced by the hydrodynamic condition being used in the bioprocess.

5.4 Requirements

- N_2 cylinder
- Conical flask
- O_2 cylinder

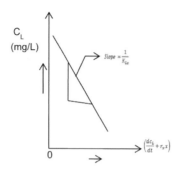

Figure 5.2 Plot for the determination of $k_L a$.

- Measuring cylinder
- Stopwatch
- Weight balance
- Fermenter: Biozenik
- Shaking incubator
- DO probe: Mettler Toledo

5.4.1 Medium

Type: Complex medium, pH $= 6.4$

Components: Yeast extract $= 4$ g/L

Peptone $= 10$ g/L

Working volume $= 2$ L

Dextrose $= 10$ g/L

5.4.2 Medium Preparation Procedure

(1) Conical flask is filled with 1 L water.

(2) To the conical flask containing water, 20 g of dextrose is added.

(3) Similarly, 20 g of peptone and 3 g of yeast extract are weighed and added to it.

(4) Water (distilled) is added to make the volume up to 1.8 L.

(5) The mouth of the conical flask is sealed with cotton plug.

(6) The prepared medium is autoclaved at 15 psi, 121°C for 15 min.

(7) After autoclaving, the medium is allowed to cool.

5.4.3 Culture Preparation

(1) Yeast culture is grown on an agar plate and stored at 4°C.
(2) One loop of culture is taken and added to the YPD medium in laminar hood to avoid contamination.
(3) The culture and medium are kept at 30°C in a shaking incubator for about 10 h. Pre-inoculum is ready for use.
(4) To 1.3 L of YPD medium, 200 mL of the grown culture is added to make the total volume up to 2 L.
(5) The culture and medium are kept at 30°C for about 6–8 h in a shaking incubator and are then transferred to the fermenter. These steps are followed to skip the lag phase, and all the cells in the fermenter are actively growing in the log phase.

5.4.4 Procedure

(1) The fermenter contains the medium.
(2) The DO probe is calibrated by sparging N_2 unsteady of O_2. N_2 acts as O_2 scavenger, and DO percentage keeps on decreasing. When the reading gets fixed, it is set to zero.
(3) The N_2 sparger is turned off, and the air sparger is turned on. The DO percentage keeps on increasing and attains a stable value. It is then set to 100.
(4) The medium is then inoculated with 5% (v/v) of inoculum previously prepared in a shake flask.
(5) The air sparger is turned on. After a steady-state condition is reached, the air is turned off. The DO of the fermentation medium is recorded at fixed intervals of time. This is continued before the critical DO is reached. It is followed by air turned on, and DO concentration is monitored.
(6) Samples are drawn out along with air. By this the valve of r_x can be calculated. When air is on, we get different values of $\left(\frac{dc_L}{dt}\right)$ at different time intervals.
(7) The sample procedure is repeated for different agitation speeds, and the change in DO percentage is recorded. The DO is monitored at 10 s intervals.

5.5 Observation

Table 5.1   Change in DO concentration in the fermentation broth after air off (given $C^* = 9$ mg/L)

Air off time (s)	Percentage of DO at different rpm		
	200	300	400
0	62.7	80.6	
10	62.6	80.1	
20	62	78.6	
30	61.1	76.9	
40	60	75	
50	58.8	73.4	
60	57.3	71.6	
70	55.8	69.9	
80	54.3	68.2	
90	52.9	66.4	
100	51.4	64.8	
110	49.8	62.3	
120	48.2	61.3	
130	46.8	59.6	
140	45.2	58	
150	43.6	56.6	
160	41.8	55.1	
170	40.3	53.7	
180	38.7	52.2	
190	36.9	50.6	77.5
200	35.4	49.1	76.3
210	34	47.6	75.3
220	32.6	46.2	75.1
230	31	45.8	74
240	29.6	44.9	73.1
250	27.6	43.7	72.6
260	26.4	42.3	71.7
270	25	41	70.9
280	23.6	39.5	70.3
290	22.4	38.2	69.6
300	21.2	36.7	68.7
310	21	35.6	68
320	21.3	34.2	67.5
330	22.2	33	66.5
340	23.3	32.1	65.9
350	24.3	30.7	65.3
360	25.1	29.7	64.7
370	25.9	28.5	63.9
380	26.7	27.6	63.4
390	28	29	62.4
400	29.2	34.3	61.9
410	30.2	37.3	61.3

Table 5.2 Change in DO concentration in the fermentation broth after air on (given $C^* = 9$ mg/L)

Air on time (s)	Percentage of DO at different rpm		
	200	300	400
420	31.6	40.9	60.6
430	33.7	43.5	60.1
440	35.6	46.2	59.3
450	36.5	48.3	58.7
460	37.5	50.3	58.2
470	38.2	52.3	57.6
480	39	54.2	57
490	39.8	55.8	56.2
500	40.7	57.4	55.7
510	41.2	58.6	56.2
520	41.8	60	55.3
530	42.9	61.5	54.8
540	44	62.5	53.6
550	44.6	63.5	53.2
560	45	65.8	50.4
570	45.3	66.6	51.5
580	45.7	67.4	50.4
590	46	68.3	50
600	46.5	69	49.5
610	—	69.6	50.4
620	—	70.3	50
630	—	70.8	49.5
640	—	71.4	49.1
650	—	71.3	52.3
660	—	71.2	56.5
670	—	72.6	60.9
680	—	72.6	65
690	—	73	69
700	—	73.5	71.7
710	—	73.7	74.9
720	—	74	77.5
730	—	74.2	79.7
740	—	74.3	81.6
750	—	74.5	83.1
760	—	74.6	84.3
770	—	75.1	85.7
780	—	75.3	86.9
790	—	75.5	87.8
800	—	75.6	89.5
810	—	78.7	90.1
820	—	—	90.4

Table 5.3 Calculated data at different rotational speed of the agitator

			200 rpm	
Time (s)	**DO (%)**	C_L **(mg/L)**	dC_L/dt **(mg/L s)**	$(dC_L/dt + Q_{O_2}x)$
0	62.7	5.643	0	0
10	62.6	5.634	−0.003	0.01015
20	62	5.580	−0.007	0.00655
30	61.1	5.499	−0.009	0.00430
40	60	5.400	−0.010	0.00295
50	58.8	5.292	−0.012	0.00115
60	57.3	5.157	−0.014	−0.00020
70	55.8	5.022	−0.014	−0.00020
80	54.3	4.887	−0.013	0.00025
90	52.9	4.761	−0.013	0.00025
100	51.4	4.626	−0.014	−0.00065
110	49.8	4.482	−0.014	−0.00110
120	48.2	4.338	−0.014	−0.00020
130	46.8	4.212	−0.014	−0.00020
140	45.2	4.068	−0.014	−0.00110
150	43.6	3.924	−0.015	−0.00200
160	41.8	3.762	−0.015	−0.00155
170	40.3	3.627	−0.014	−0.00065
180	38.7	3.483	−0.015	−0.00200
190	36.9	3.321	−0.015	−0.00155
200	35.4	3.186	−0.013	0.00025
210	34	3.060	−0.013	0.00070
220	32.6	2.934	−0.014	−0.00020
230	31	2.790	−0.014	−0.00020
240	29.6	2.664	−0.014	−0.00065
250	27.9	2.511	−0.014	−0.00110
260	26.4	2.376	−0.013	0.00025
270	25	2.250	−0.013	0.00070
280	23.6	2.124	−0.012	0.00160
290	22.4	2.016	−0.011	0.00250
300	21.2	1.908	−0.006	0.00700
310	21	1.890	0.000	0.01375
320	21.3	1.917	0.005	0.01870
330	22.2	1.998	0.009	0.02230
340	23.3	2.097	0.009	0.02275
350	24.3	2.187	0.010	0.02320
360	25.5	2.295	0.011	0.02410
370	26.7	2.403	0.011	0.02455
380	28	2.520	0.011	0.02455
390	29.2	2.628	0.010	0.02320

Table 5.3 (*Continued*)

Time (s)	DO (%)	C_L (mg/L)	dC_L/dt (mg/L s)	$(dC_L/dt + Q_{O_2}x)$
		200 rpm		
400	30.2	2.718	0.011	0.02410
410	31.6	2.844	0.016	0.02905
420	33.7	3.033	0.013	0.02635
430	34.5	3.105	0.009	0.02185
440	35.6	3.204	0.009	0.02230
450	36.5	3.285	0.009	0.02185
460	37.5	3.375	0.008	0.02095
470	38.2	3.438	0.007	0.02005
480	39	3.510	0.007	0.02050
490	39.8	3.582	0.008	0.02095
500	40.7	3.663	0.006	0.01960
510	41.2	3.708	0.005	0.01825
520	41.8	3.762	0.005	0.01870
530	42.4	3.816	0.005	0.01825
540	42.9	3.861	0.007	0.02050
550	44	3.960	0.008	0.02095
560	44.6	4.014	0.004	0.01780
570	45	4.050	0.003	0.01645
580	45.3	4.077	0.003	0.01645
590	45.7	4.113	0.003	0.01645
600	46	4.140	0.004	0.01690
610	46.5	4.185	−0.207	−0.19370
		300 rpm		
0	80.6	7.254		
10	80.1	7.209	−0.009	0.00430
20	78.6	7.074	−0.014	−0.00110
30	76.9	6.921	−0.016	−0.00290
40	75	6.750	−0.016	−0.00245
50	73.4	6.606	−0.015	−0.00200
60	71.6	6.444	−0.016	−0.00245
70	69.9	6.291	−0.015	−0.00200
80	68.2	6.138	−0.016	−0.00245
90	66.4	5.976	−0.015	−0.00200
100	64.8	5.832	−0.016	−0.00290
110	62.8	5.652	−0.016	−0.00245
120	61.3	5.517	−0.014	−0.00110
130	59.6	5.364	−0.015	−0.00155
140	58	5.220	−0.014	−0.00020
150	56.6	5.094	−0.013	0.00025

(*Contd.*)

Table 5.3 (*Continued*)

Time (s)	DO (%)	C_L (mg/L)	dC_L/dt (mg/L s)	$(dC_L/dt + Q_{O_2}x)$
		300 rpm		
160	55.1	4.959	−0.013	0.00025
170	53.7	4.833	−0.013	0.00025
180	52.2	4.698	−0.014	−0.00065
190	50.6	4.554	−0.014	−0.00065
200	49.1	4.419	−0.014	−0.00020
210	47.6	4.284	−0.013	0.00025
220	46.2	4.158	−0.013	0.00070
230	44.8	4.032	−0.011	0.00205
240	43.7	3.933	−0.011	0.00205
250	42.3	3.807	−0.012	0.00115
260	41	3.690	−0.013	0.00070
270	39.5	3.555	−0.013	0.00070
280	38.2	3.438	−0.013	0.00070
290	36.7	3.303	−0.012	0.00160
300	35.6	3.204	−0.011	0.00205
310	34.2	3.078	−0.012	0.00160
320	33	2.970	−0.009	0.00385
330	32.1	2.889	−0.010	0.00295
340	30.7	2.763	−0.011	0.00250
350	29.7	2.673	−0.010	0.00340
360	28.5	2.565	−0.009	0.00385
370	27.6	2.484	0.002	0.01555
380	29	2.610	0.018	0.03175
390	31.7	2.853	0.026	0.03940
400	34.8	3.132	0.027	0.04075
410	37.8	3.402	0.027	0.04075
420	40.9	3.681	0.026	0.03895
430	43.5	3.915	0.024	0.03715
440	46.2	4.158	0.022	0.03490
450	48.3	4.347	0.018	0.03175
460	50.3	4.527	0.018	0.03130
470	52.3	4.707	0.018	0.03085
480	54.2	4.878	0.016	0.02905
490	55.8	5.022	0.014	0.02770
500	57.4	5.166	0.013	0.02590
510	58.6	5.274	0.012	0.02500
520	60	5.400	0.013	0.02635
530	61.5	5.535	0.011	0.02455
540	62.5	5.625	0.009	0.02230
550	63.5	5.715	0.009	0.02275

Table 5.3 (*Continued*)

		300 rpm		
Time (s)	**DO (%)**	C_L **(mg/L)**	dC_L/dt **(mg/L s)**	$(dC_L/dt + Q_{O_2}x)$
560	64.6	5.814	0.010	0.02365
570	65.8	5.922	0.009	0.02230
580	66.6	5.994	0.007	0.02050
590	67.4	6.066	0.008	0.02095
600	68.3	6.147	0.007	0.02050
610	69	6.210	0.006	0.01915
620	69.6	6.264	0.006	0.01915
630	70.3	6.327	0.005	0.01870
640	70.8	6.372	0.005	0.01825
650	71.4	6.426	0.004	0.01780
660	71.8	6.462	0.004	0.01690
670	72.2	6.498	0.004	0.01690
680	72.6	6.534	0.004	0.01690
690	73	6.570	0.004	0.01735
700	73.5	6.615	0.003	0.01645
710	73.7	6.633	0.002	0.01555
720	74	6.660	0.002	0.01555
730	74.2	6.678	0.001	0.01465
740	74.3	6.687	0.001	0.01465
750	74.5	6.705	0.001	0.01465
760	74.6	6.714	0.003	0.01600
770	75.1	6.759	0.003	0.01645
780	75.3	6.777	0.002	0.01510
790	75.5	6.795	0.001	0.01465
800	75.6	6.804	0.001	0.01420
810	75.7	6.813	−0.340	−0.32690
		400 rpm		
0	98	8.820	0.000	0.00000
10	97.2	8.748	−0.008	−0.00120
20	96.2	8.658	−0.010	−0.00345
30	94.9	8.541	−0.013	−0.00570
40	93.4	8.406	−0.014	−0.00660
50	91.9	8.271	−0.012	−0.00480
60	90.8	8.172	−0.010	−0.00345
70	89.6	8.064	−0.012	−0.00480
80	88.2	7.938	−0.010	−0.00345
90	87.3	7.857	−0.010	−0.00300
100	86	7.740	−0.010	−0.00300
110	85.1	7.659	−0.009	−0.00210

(*Contd.*)

Table 5.3   (*Continued*)

	400 rpm			
Time (s)	DO (%)	C_L (mg/L)	dC_L/dt (mg/L s)	$(dC_L/dt + Q_{O_2}x)$
120	84	7.560	−0.009	−0.00255
130	83	7.470	−0.009	−0.00165
140	82.1	7.389	−0.009	−0.00165
150	81.1	7.299	−0.009	−0.00165
160	80.2	7.218	−0.008	−0.00120
170	79.3	7.137	−0.008	−0.00120
180	78.4	7.056	−0.008	−0.00120
190	77.5	6.975	−0.007	−0.00030
200	76.8	6.912	−0.008	−0.00075
210	75.8	6.822	−0.008	−0.00075
220	75.1	6.759	−0.008	−0.00120
230	74	6.660	−0.009	−0.00210
240	73.1	6.579	−0.006	0.00060
250	72.6	6.534	−0.006	0.00060
260	71.7	6.453	−0.008	−0.00075
270	70.9	6.381	−0.006	0.00060
280	70.3	6.327	−0.006	0.00105
290	69.6	6.264	−0.007	−0.00030
300	68.7	6.183	−0.007	−0.00030
310	68	6.120	−0.005	0.00150
320	67.5	6.075	−0.007	0.00015
330	66.5	5.985	−0.007	−0.00030
340	65.9	5.931	−0.005	0.00150
350	65.3	5.877	−0.005	0.00150
360	64.7	5.823	−0.006	0.00060
370	63.9	5.751	−0.006	0.00105
380	63.4	5.706	−0.007	0.00015
390	62.4	5.616	−0.007	0.00015
400	61.9	5.571	−0.005	0.00195
410	61.3	5.517	−0.006	0.00105
420	60.6	5.454	−0.005	0.00150
430	60.1	5.409	−0.006	0.00105
440	59.3	5.337	−0.006	0.00060
450	58.7	5.283	−0.005	0.00195
460	58.2	5.238	−0.005	0.00195
470	57.6	5.184	−0.005	0.00150
470	470	5.130	−0.006	0.00060
480	480	5.058	−0.006	0.00105
490	490	5.013	−0.004	0.00285
500	500	4.977	−0.004	0.00285

Table 5.3 (*Continued*)

		400 rpm		
Time (s)	DO (%)	C_L (mg/L)	dC_L/dt (mg/L s)	$(dC_L/dt + Q_{O_2}x)$
510	510	4.932	−0.008	−0.00075
520	520	4.824	−0.007	−0.00030
530	530	4.788	−0.005	0.00195
540	540	4.725	−0.005	0.00150
550	550	4.680	−0.004	0.00240
560	560	4.635	−0.007	−0.00030
570	570	4.536	−0.007	0.00015
580	580	4.500	−0.004	0.00285
590	590	4.455	−0.004	0.00285
600	600	4.419	−0.004	0.00285
610	610	4.374	−0.004	0.00285
620	620	4.338	0.002	0.00915
630	630	4.419	0.018	0.02535
640	640	4.707	0.033	0.04020
650	650	5.085	0.039	0.04560
660	660	5.481	0.038	0.04515
670	670	5.850	0.036	0.04335
680	680	6.210	0.030	0.03705
690	690	6.453	0.027	0.03345
700	700	6.741	0.026	0.03300
710	710	6.975	0.022	0.02850
720	720	7.173	0.018	0.02535
730	730	7.344	0.015	0.02220
740	740	7.479	0.012	0.01905
750	750	7.587	0.012	0.01860
760	760	7.713	0.012	0.01860
770	770	7.821	0.009	0.01635
780	780	7.902	0.009	0.01545
790	790	7.992	0.008	0.01455
800	800	8.055	0.006	0.01275
810	810	8.109	−0.403	−0.39585

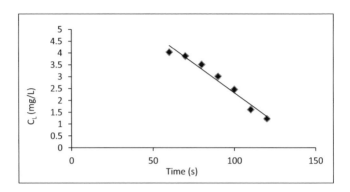

Figure 5.3   DO profile during air off at 200 rpm.

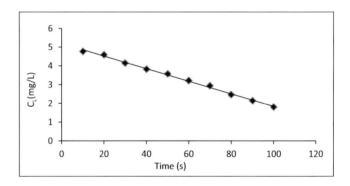

Figure 5.4   DO profile during air off at 300 rpm.

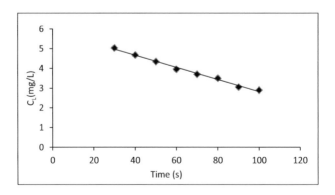

Figure 5.5   DO profile during air off at 400 rpm.

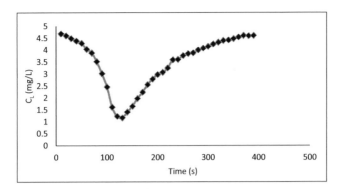

Figure 5.6 DO profile during air off and air on at 200 rpm.

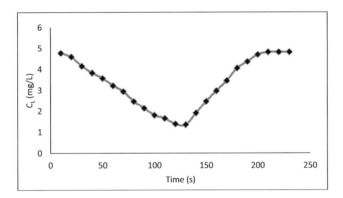

Figure 5.7 DO profile during air off and air on at 300 rpm.

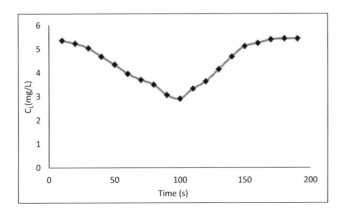

Figure 5.8 DO profile during air off and air on at 400 rpm.

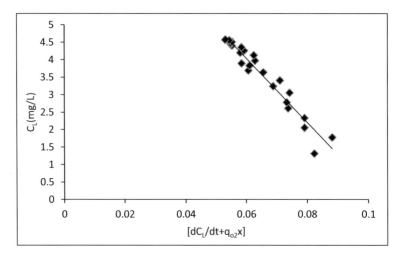

Figure 5.9   Plot of c_L versus $(\frac{dc_L}{dt} + q_{O_2}\, x)$ at 200 rpm.

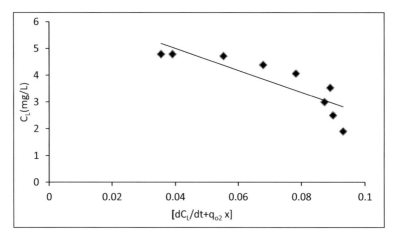

Figure 5.10   Plot of c_L versus $(\frac{dc_L}{dt} + q_{O_2}\, x)$ at 300 rpm.

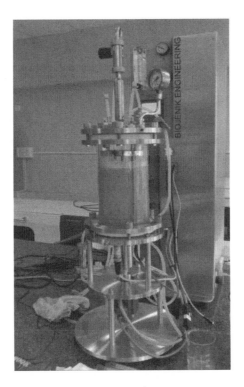

Figure 5.11   Plot of c_L versus $\left(\frac{dc_L}{dt} + q_{O_2}x\right)$ at 400 rpm.

5.5.1 Sample Calculations

(1) For 300 rpm

From plot of C_L versus time (air off)

Slope $q_{O_2}x = 0.0133$

$q_{O_2}x = 0.0133$, $x = 680$ mg/L

$\Rightarrow q_{O_2} = \dfrac{0.0133}{680} = 0.00001956\,\text{s}^{-1} = 1.956 \times 10^{-5}\,\text{s}^{-1}$

From plot of C_L versus $\left[\dfrac{dc_L}{dt} + q_{O_2}x\right]$

Slope $= \dfrac{-1}{k_L a} = -147.53$

$\Rightarrow k_L a = 6.773 \times 10^{-3}\,\text{s}^{-1}$

(2) For 400 rpm

From plot of C_L versus time (air off)

Slope $= q_{O_2}x = 0.0133$, $x = 960$ mg/L

$$q_{O_2} = \frac{0.0133}{960} = 1.385 \times 10^{-5} s^{-1}$$

From plot of C_L versus $\left[\dfrac{dc_L}{dt} + q_{O_2}x \right]$

Slope $= \dfrac{-1}{k_L a} = -131.95$

$k_L a = 7.579 \times 10^{-3} s^{-1}$

(3) For 500 rpm

From plot of C_L versus time (air off)

Slope $= q_{O_2}x = 0.0069$

$q_{O_2} \times 1170$ mg/L $= 0.0069$

$q_{O_2} = 5.9 \times 10^{-6} s^{-1}$

From plot of C_L versus $\left[\dfrac{dc_L}{dt} + q_{O_2}x \right]$

Slope $= \dfrac{-1}{k_L a} = -57.361$

$k_L a = 0.017433\ s^{-1}$

Table 5.4 Calculated data

Rotational speed (rpm)	q_{O_2} (s^{-1})	$K_L a\,(s^{-1})$
300	1.956×10^{-5}	0.006778
400	1.385×10^{-5}	0.007579
500	5.9×10^{-6}	0.017433

5.6 Discussion

The measurement of $k_L a$ provides important information about a bioprocess or bioreactor. $k_L a$ ensures that processing conditions should be maintained such that an adequate supply of oxygen is available for the proliferation of cells. The k_La value can also be used to optimize control variables over the life cycle of a bioprocess. Such optimizations would be based on the oxygen demand at various points in the process and the growth phase of an organism. The criteria for optimization would be product yield, power consumption, or processing time.

5.6.1 Importance of k_La Value

- **New equipment:** Measurement of k_La is made for evaluating new reactor designs, new gas sparging equipment, and/or operating conditions to confirm the suitability of the process for microbial growth.
- **Process optimization:** In scale-up and manufacturing situations, measuring k_La is a key to control oxygenation at the optimum rate.
- **Relevance to a single-use bioreactor:** The ranges of k_La values that a single-use bioreactor can support, coupled with the operating conditions required to achieve those ranges, are fundamental in the selection of reactor equipment.

5.6.2 Benefits of Measuring k_La

- Assurance that biological growth is not impeded by inadequate oxygen concentration.
- Better ability to find out the time for the attainment of the DO concentration for optimal processing.
- Prevention of wasted energy and cost associated with unnecessarily high oxygen concentrations.

5.6.3 Parameters Influencing k_La Value

- **Pressure:** As pressure increases, the movement or diffusion of oxygen becomes very difficult as diffusivity decreases. So k_La is also decreased.
- **Temperature:** As temperature increases, air diffusion decreases, thus decreasing the mass transfer rate.

- **Size and cell type:** As the size of cells increases, the uptake of oxygen increases. So $k_L a$ also increases.
- **Foaming:** Foam formation occurs due to air sparging through protein-containing components in the medium. This foam may chock valves or cause contamination. To prevent this, one can use antifoaming agents, but these should be added only in the desired amount as these may affect the values of $k_L a$.
- **Agitation speed:** The more the agitation speed, the shorter the time to reach the saturated level of DO concentration. So $k_L a$ increases.
- **Composition of medium:** The medium contains carbon source, nitrogen source, minerals, vitamins, and other elements in trace amounts. The variation in their concentration may also affect the $k_L a$ value.

5.7 Conclusion

The volumetric mass transfer coefficient ($k_L a$) increases as the rotational speed of the stirrer increases from 300 rpm to 500 rpm. This indicates improvement in the rate of mass transfer, which may be due to the disintegration of air bubbles at higher rotational speed of the stirrer, which increases the surface area.

References

1. Bailey, J. E. and Ollis, D. F., *Biochemical Engineering Fundamentals*, McGraw-Hill Inc., New Delhi, India, 2010.
2. Doran, P. M., *Bioprocess Engineering Principles*, Second Edition, Academic Press, Waltham, USA, 2012.
3. Aiba, S., Humphrey, A. E., and Millis, N. F., *Biochemical Engineering*, Academic Press, USA, 1973.
4. Das, D. and Das, D., *Biochemical Engineering: An Introductory Textbook*, Jenny Stanford Publishing, Singapore, 2019.

Experiment 6

Mixing Time Determination

Objective: To correlate the mixing time with the power drawn by the agitator

6.1 Purpose

To determine the mixing time and to find out its correlation with the Reynolds number

6.2 Theory

Mixing is a physical process that aims at reducing nonuniformities in fluids by eliminating gradient of concentration, temperature, and other properties associated with reaction in the bioreactor. The performance of a bioreactor depends on the mixing characteristics of the medium.

Mixing time is the time required from the start of mixing operation to the time when terminal mixing is achieved. Terminal mixing is a specific degree of mixing achieved at the time when uniformity of the composition in the specified sample size is

Biochemical Engineering: A Laboratory Manual
Debabrata Das and Debayan Das
Copyright © 2021 Jenny Stanford Publishing Pte. Ltd.
ISBN 978-981-4877-36-7 (Hardcover), 978-1-003-11105-4 (eBook)
www.jennystanford.com

not further changed by additional mixing within the precision of the instrumentation used, i.e., homogeneity of the fermentation medium. Mixing time can be measured by injecting a tracer into the bioreactor and following the change in a particular parameter with the change in time.

Commonly used tracers include acid, base, and concentrated salt solution. The corresponding detectors are pH probes and conductivity cells. It can also be measured by tracing the temperature response after the addition of a small quantity of heated liquid.

6.2.1 Mechanism of Mixing

For effective mixing, fluid circulated by the impeller must sweep the entire vessel in a reasonable time. Also the velocity of the fluid leaving the impeller must be sufficient to carry the material into the most remote parts of the reactor.

The mixing process can be described as a combination of three physical processes: distribution, dispersion, and diffusion.

6.2.1.1 Distribution

The process whereby materials are transported to all regions of the vessel by bulk circulation of the fluid is known as distribution. It is often the slowest step in the mixing process. Factors affecting distribution are the size of the circulation path, time taken to traverse the path, and regularity of liquid pumping at the impeller.

6.2.1.2 Dispersion

Dispersion is the process of breaking up bulk flow into smaller and smaller eddies (regions of rotational flow). It facilitates rapid transfer of materials throughout the vessel. The degree of homogeneity as a result of dispersion is limited by the size of the smallest eddies, which may be formed in a particular fluid.

6.2.1.3 Diffusion

Ever in turbulent medium, the region closest to the phase boundary is mostly a thin stagnant film. Mixing in those regions mostly takes place by molecular diffusion.

6.2.1.4 Common stirrers

Mixing can be of two types based on the direction of motion of the impeller:

(1) **Axial:** movement of fluid in the vertical direction, along the axis.
(2) **Radial:** movement of fluid along the radius of the reactor, parallel to the axis.

Impeller is a rotating component of a centrifugal pump, which transfers energy from the motor that drives the pump to the fluid being pumped by accelerating the fluid outward from the center of rotation. It is usually made of iron, steel, bronze, brass, aluminum, or plastic. Depending on geometry, there are various types of impellers that have significant difference in the type of rotational motion they cause (Fig. 6.1).

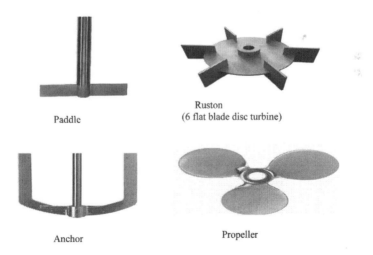

Paddle

Ruston
(6 flat blade disc turbine)

Anchor

Propeller

Figure 6.1 Different stirrers used for mixing in liquid.

6.2.1.5 Power consumption

Electrical power is used to drive impellers in a stirred tank. For a particular speed, the power requirement depends on the resistance offered by the fluid to the rotation of the impeller. Friction in the stirrer motor gearbox and seal reduces the energy transmitted to the fluid; therefore, the electrical power consumed by the stirrer motor is always greater than the mixing power by an amount depending on the efficiency of the drive. Energy costs for the operation of stirrer in bioreactors are an important consideration in process economics.

The movement of the liquid inside the bioreactor is due to the agitator rotation. The normal Reynolds number indicates the flow characteristics of the fluid. This is expressed as

$$N_{Re} = \frac{D_i\, u\, \rho}{\mu} \tag{6.1}$$

where D_i is the diameter of the impeller or agitator, u is the velocity of the fluid, ρ is the density of the fluid, and μ is the viscosity of the fluid.

In the case of a bioreactor, the circular movement of the liquid is due to the movement of the stirrer. Here the flow characteristics of the liquid are expressed as the agitator Reynolds number. The rotational velocity of the liquid can be expressed as

$$u = n\pi D_i \tag{6.2}$$

where n is the rotational speed of the stirrer.

If we put the value of u in Eq. 6.1, we get

$$N_{Re} = \frac{D_i\, n\, \pi\, D_i\, \rho}{\mu} = \frac{\pi\, n\, D_i^2\, \rho}{\mu} \tag{6.3}$$

One can write

$$N_{Re} \propto \frac{n\, D_i^2\, \rho}{\mu} \tag{6.4}$$

Again, the power drawn by the agitator can be expressed as

$$P = N_P n^3 D_i^5 \rho$$

where P is the power in watts, and N_P is the power number [2–4].

The value of the power number depends on the Reynolds number.

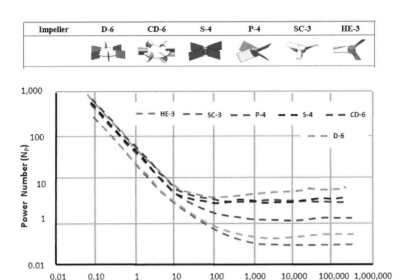

Figure 6.2 Correlation between the power number and the agitator Reynolds number (N_{Re}) using different types of agitators (taken from the Ph.D. thesis of Zheng Ma [1]).

6.3 Apparatus Required

- Fermenter: Bioengineering AG KLF 2000
- pH probe: Mettle Toledo
- Syringe
- Stopwatch
- Controlling unit

6.4 Preparation of CMC Solution

Carboxymethyl cellulose (CMC): 5 g/L

$$\text{Structure: } (C_6H_{10}O_5)_n - CH_2 - COOH$$

CMC is used because the media should be chosen such that the composition of the media should not change on the addition of acid or alkali. Also the flow characteristics (viscosity, density, etc.) of CMC are similar to those of the fermentation medium.

Working volume $= 2$ L

Amount of CMC to be added $= 10$ g

1 N 35% HCL: 13.5 mL of acid $+ 136.5$ mL distilled water

1 N NaOH: 40 g in 50 mL distilled water

CMC is sparingly soluble in water. The following procedure is followed for the solubilization of CMC in water:

(1) To 1 L of distilled water in a conical flask, 5 g of CMC is added and is heated with continuous stirring.
(2) After all the CMC in the solution dissolves, again 5 g of CMC is added with 1 L water.
(3) The mixture is continuously heated along with constant stirring to facilitate the dissolving process.
(4) Due to the heating of the solution, water gets evaporated. Hence, the required amount of distilled water is added to the make the resulting volume up to 2 L.
(5) The resulting CMC solution is allowed to cool before transferring to the fermenter.

6.5 Mixing Time Determination

(1) The CMC solution is added to the fermenter via the feed port.
(2) The controlling unit of the fermenter is turned on. The pH probe is connected to the control unit and is inserted in the fermenter vessel. Temperature is $35.3°$C, and initial pH is 6.36.
(3) The agitation speed is set to 100 rpm. To the reactor, 1 mL of 1 N NaOH is added, and the stopwatch is started. As soon as one obtains a stable pH value, the stopwatch is stopped and the time is recorded.

(4) Now 1 mL of 1 N HCL is added, and the stopwatch is started and is stopped when the control unit displays a stable pH value.

(5) The same process is repeated for agitation speeds of 200 rpm to 500 rpm, and the corresponding mixing time is noted down.

6.6 Observation

Table 6.1 Mixing time at different agitation speeds

Agitation speed (rpm)	Test number	Mixing time (s)		Overall average mixing time (s)
		Acid	Base	
100	1	140	135	141.25
	2	150	140	
	Average t_m(s)	145	137.5	
200	1	90	100	95
	2	95	95	
	Average t_m	92.5	97.5	
300	1	79	79	78.25
	2	80	75	
	Average t_m	79.5	77	
400	1	54	53	56.5
	2	60	59	
	Average t_m	57	56	
500	1	48	51	48
	2	50	43	
	Average t_m	49	47	
600	1	43	45	45
	2	45	47	
	Average t_m	44	46	

Assume the following values:

Density of CMC solution, $\rho = 1000$ kg/m^3 and μ (viscosity) $= 0.5$ kg/m s

Diameter of impeller $(D_i) = 5.5$ cm $= 0.055$ m

Table 6.2   Calculated data

Agitator speed (rpm)	Power number (N_p)	Power consumption (P) (watts)	Agitator Reynolds number (N_{Re})
100	7	0.01631	10.0833
200	5	0.0932	20.1667
300	4.1	0.2579	30.250
400	3.7	0.5518	40.33
500	3.5	1.0194	50.4167
600	3.3	1.6608	60.50

6.7 Sample Calculation

The agitator Reynolds number (N_{Re}) is

$$N_{Re} = \frac{n \times D_i^2 \times \rho}{\mu}$$

where n is the agitator speed (rps), D_i is the diameter of the impeller (m), ρ is the density, and μ is the viscosity.

Here

$$n = 100 \, \text{rpm} = \left(\frac{100}{60}\right) \text{rps}$$

$D_1 = 0.055$ m, density (ρ) $= 1000$ kg/m^3, viscosity (μ) $= 0.5$ kg/m s

$$N_{Re} = \left(\frac{100}{60}\right) \times \frac{(0.055)^2 \times 1000}{0.5} = 10.0833$$

Power consumption by the agitator is

$$P = N_P n^3 D_1^5 \rho$$

where P is the power, N_p is the power number, n is the agitator speed (rps), D_1 is the impeller diameter (m), and ρ is the density.

At $n = 100 \, \text{rpm} = \left(\frac{100}{60}\right)$ rps, $N_P = 7$.

$$P = 7 \times \left(\frac{100}{60}\right)^3 \times (0.055)^5 \times 1000$$

$$= 0.0163 \, \text{kgm}^2/\text{s}^3$$

$$= 0.0163 \, \text{W}$$

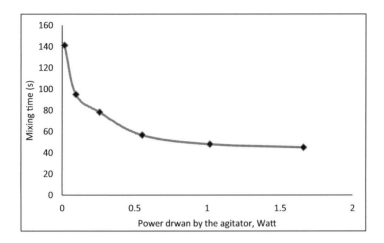

Figure 6.3   Plot of mixing time versus power drawn by the agitator.

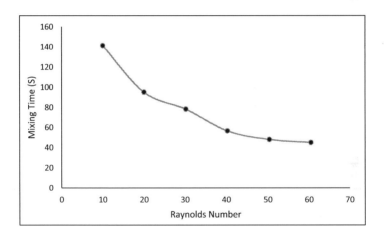

Figure 6.4   Plot of mixing time versus agitator Reynolds number.

6.8 Result and Discussion

The minimum mixing time is 45 s (overall average) at the agitator speed of 500 rpm. The power consumption at 500 rpm is $P = 1.02$ W.

From the experimental data obtained, it can be clearly deduced that as one increases the impeller speed, the mixing time decreases. Power consumption strongly depends on stirrer diameter and stirrer speed. Small changes in impeller size have a large effect on the power requirements.

The design of an industry-scale bioprocess is usually based on the performance of a small-scale prototype. Mixing is an important function of bioreactors, so it should be taken into consideration during scale-up. However, an increase in stirrer speed also enhances the power consumption. As the volume of mixing vessels is increased to keep the mixing time constant, the velocity of fluid in the tank must be increased in proportion to the size.

Instead of mixing time, P/V is kept constant during scale-up. Reduced productivity and performance often accompany scale-up of bioreactors as a result of lower mixing efficiency and subsequent alteration of the physical environment. Another way of improving design procedure is to use scale-down methods. Scale experiments to determine operating parameters are carried under conditions that can be actually realized, physically and economically, at the production scale.

Mixing can be improved by changing the configuration of the vessel. Baffles should be installed. These are attached to the stirrer fermenter and produce greater turbulence. For efficient mixing, the impeller should be mounted below the geometric center of the vessel. Mixing is facilitated when the circulation current below the impeller is smaller than that above. Fluid particles leaving the impeller at the same time then take different periods of time to return and exchange materials.

Another method for improving mixing is using multiple impellers although this requires an increase in power input. Effective mixing in tall fermenters requires more than one impeller. Mixing in bioreactors must provide the shear condition necessary to disperse bubble droplets and cell flow. Hydrodynamic effects must be studied because shear damage is a significant problem in large-scale culture.

6.9 Conclusion

- Mixing time decreases as we increase the agitator speed of impeller. It becomes constant after a particular impeller speed or Reynolds number.
- Power consumption also increases with the agitator speed. This is to be optimized.

References

1. Ma, Z., Impeller power draw across the full Reynolds number spectrum, Ph.D. Thesis, University of Dayton, 2014.
2. Das, D. and Das, D., *Biochemical Engineering: An Introductory Textbook*, Jenny Stanford Publishing, Singapore, 2019.
3. Bailey, J. E. and Ollis, D. F., *Biochemical Engineering Fundamentals*, McGraw-Hill Inc., New Delhi, India, 2010.
4. Doran, P. M., *Bioprocess Engineering Principles*, Second Edition, Academic Press, Waltham, USA, 2012.

Experiment 7

Determination of Air Filter Efficiency

Objective: To find out the effectiveness of air filter

7.1 Purpose

To determine the effectiveness of air filter using glass wool fiber

7.2 Theory

The mechanism of collection of aerosol particles by fibrous media may be classified as follows:

- Inertial impaction
- Interception
- Diffusion
- Settling by gravitational force
- Electrostatic force

Settling by gravitational force in the case of fibrous filters may be neglected because the diameter of the particles to be collected is in the order of 1 μm. Again it is expected that charged organisms would be more effectively collected than neutral ones. It has been

Biochemical Engineering: A Laboratory Manual
Debabrata Das and Debayan Das
Copyright © 2021 Jenny Stanford Publishing Pte. Ltd.
ISBN 978-981-4877-36-7 (Hardcover), 978-1-003-11105-4 (eBook)
www.jennystanford.com

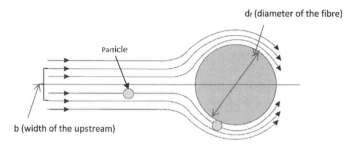

Figure 7.1 Air flow is perpendicular against the cross section of the fiber (Das and Das, 2019).

found that *Bacillus subtilis* possesses 70% positive, 15% negative, and 15% neutral charge. However, there is little quantitative data available to find out the contribution of the electrostatic charge of the microorganisms to the overall collection efficiency of the fibrous air sterilization filter. So the first three mechanisms—inertial impaction, interception, and diffusion—are considered in detail.

It is assumed that

(1) Single cylindrical fibers are placed perpendicularly to the aerosol flow in an infinite space, and that the air flow around the cylinder is laminar with no vortices.

(2) The following analyses are two dimensional, as shown in Fig. 7.1.

7.2.1 Inertial Impaction

The flow pattern of the particles deviates from that of the air flow due to the inertia of the particles as they approach the cylindrical surface. In Fig. 7.1, the width of the upstream air flow is denoted by b. Particles that move in the streamlines of air beyond b will not touch the cylinder surface even after they deviate from the air streamline near the cylinder. Then the collection efficiency of a single fiber due to the inertial effect of the particles is

$$\eta_0' = \frac{b}{d_f} \tag{7.1}$$

$\eta_0' = 0$, when $\varphi = \dfrac{1}{16}$

where

$$\varphi = \text{inertial parameter} = \frac{C\,\rho_p\,d_p^2\,V_o}{18\mu\,d_f} \qquad (7.2)$$

At the critical air velocity V_c, φ is equal to 1/16.

$$V_c = (1.125)\,\frac{\mu\,d_f}{C\,\rho_p\,d_p^2} \qquad (7.3)$$

where C is Cunningham's correction factor for slip flow, ρ_p is the density of particle (g/cm^3), d_p is the particle diameter (μm, cm), d_f is the fiber diameter (μm, cm), and μ is the viscosity of air (g/cm s). At the air velocity below the value of V_c, the inertial impaction of particle may be neglected [1, 3].

7.2.2 Interception

The particles when entrained in the streamlines of air are collected by contact with the fibers. They are said to be intercepted. The streamline of air flow is at a distance of $d_p/2$ from the fiber surface. This is a limited condition for the deposition of the entrained particles as they pass a cylindrical fiber. Then, the collection efficiency due to interception may be written as

$$\eta_0'' = \frac{1}{2(2 - \ln N_{Re})}\left\{2(1 + N_R)\ln(1 + N_R) - (1 + N_R) + \frac{1}{(1 + N_R)}\right\} \qquad (7.4)$$

where $N_R = \dfrac{d_p}{d_f}$ = Geometrical ratio and

N_{Re} = Reynolds number = $\dfrac{du\rho}{\mu}$

7.2.3 Diffusion

Small particles display Brownian motion and thus may be collected on the surface of the fibers as the particles are displaced from their median center of location. If the displacement of the particle is $2X_0$, the collection efficiency due to diffusion may be written as

$$\eta_0''' = \frac{1}{2\,(2 - \ln N_{Re})}\left[2\left(1 + \frac{2X_0}{d_f}\right)\right]\ln\left(1 + \frac{2X_0}{d_f}\right)$$
$$- \left(1 + \frac{2X_0}{d_f}\right) + \frac{1}{1 + 2X_0/d_f} \tag{7.5}$$

$$\frac{2X_0}{d_f} = 1.12\frac{2\,(2 - \ln N_{Re})\,D_{BM}}{V\,d_f} \tag{7.6}$$

where $D_{BM} = C\,KT/3\pi\,\mu d_p$ = Diffusivity of the particle

7.2.4 Collection Efficiencies

Different collection efficiencies of the filter can be calculated as follows:

$$\text{Single fiber efficiency }(\eta_\alpha) = \frac{\pi\,d_f\,(1 - \alpha)}{4\,L\alpha}\ln\frac{N_1}{N_2} \tag{7.7}$$

where α is the volume fraction of the filter.

$$\text{Overall collection efficiency }(\eta_0) = \frac{\eta_\alpha}{1 + 4.5\alpha}$$
$$\text{(for } 0 < \alpha < 0.10) \tag{7.8}$$

$$\text{Collection efficiency (experimental) }(\eta) = \frac{N_1 - N_2}{N_1} \tag{7.9}$$

7.3 Materials

- Glass wool filter
- Wet gas flow meter
- Rotameter
- Test tubes
- Saline ware (0.85%)
- Nutrient agar
- Microscope
- Stopwatch

7.4 Procedure

The number of airborne microbes in the inlet and outlet is determined at different air flow rates using a plating technique containing nutrient agar. A definite volume of air is sparged in the 20 mL 0.85% w/v saline water. It was diluted depending on the concentration of the viable cells before inoculation in the Petri plates. These plates are incubated at 37°C for 2–3 days. The number of colonies present indicates the presence of viable cells.

7.5 Observation

A schematic diagram of the process is shown in Fig. 7.2.

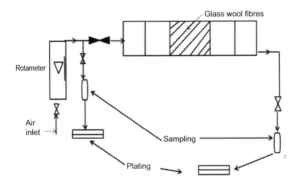

Figure 7.2 Schematic diagram of the experimental setup (Das and Das, 2019).

Diameter of the glass wool fiber is 19 μm; diameter of the air filter is 7.1 cm; cross-sectional area of the air filter is 39.57 cm²; filter thickness is 2.6 cm; and packing fraction (α) is 0.033.

7.5.1 Sample Calculations

Flow rate $= 1000$ mL/min

$$\text{Velocity} = \frac{1000}{39.57 \times 60} = 0.42 \text{ cm/s}$$

Table 7.1 Performance of the air filter

Viable bacteria input $v(N_1)$	Viable bacteria output (N_2)	Air flow rate (L/min)	Velocity of air (v) (cm/s)	Collection efficiency (η)	Single fiber efficiency (η_α)	Overall collection efficiency (η_0)
140	40	1	0.42	0.714	0.000210	0.000177
140	58	2	0.84	0.586	0.000147	0.000128
40	14	3	1.26	0.900	0.000387	0.000337
140	6	4.5	1.89	0.968	0.000529	0.000461

$$\text{Collection efficiency, } \eta = \frac{N_1 - N_2}{N_1} = \frac{140 - 40}{140} = 0.714$$

$$\text{Single fiber efficiency } (\eta_\alpha) = \frac{\pi d_f(1 - \alpha)}{4L\alpha} \ln \frac{N_1}{N_2}$$

$$= \frac{3.14 \times 19 \times 10^{-6}(1 - 0.033)}{4 \times 2.6 \times 0.033} \ln \frac{140}{40}$$

$$= 0.000210$$

$$\text{Overall collection efficiency } (\eta_0) = \frac{\eta_\alpha}{1 + 4.5\alpha} = \frac{0.000210}{1.185}$$

$$= 0.000177$$

7.6 Discussion

- In air filtration, glass wool fiber is used because it can be regenerated by sterilization.
- Jute fiber can also be used instead of glass wool fiber, but it cannot be reused again and again. After sterilization, the fiber becomes fragile, and as a result, leakage of microbes from pores can occur.
- If the fibers are not sterilized time to time, the pores become saturated, and it can also lead to contamination.
- When the velocity is less, diffusion occurs due to the Brownian movement of the particles.
- If the particle diameter is less than the pore size of the glass wool filter, the collection efficiency occurs mainly due to

interception, and for higher velocity, it occurs due to inertial impaction.

7.7 Conclusion

The collection efficiency of glass wool air filter decreases with the air velocity, which is followed by an increasing trend. A similar type of observation is also reported in the literature. The decrease in collection efficiency at low air velocity is mainly due to the diffusion phenomenon for the collection of particles. However, at higher velocity, the collection of particles is mainly due to interception and inertial impaction.

References

1. Aiba, S., Humphrey, A. E., and Millis, N. F., *Biochemical Engineering*, Academic Press, 1973.
2. Das, D. and Das, D., *Biochemical Engineering: An Introductory Textbook*, Jenny Stanford Publishing, Singapore, 1919.
3. Bailey, J. E. and Ollis, D. F., *Biochemical Engineering Fundamentals*, McGraw-Hill Inc., New Delhi, India, 2010.

Experiment 8

Kill Curve Determination

Objective: To determine the death rate constant of *Saccharomyces cerevisiae*

8.1 Purpose

To find out the death rate constant of *S. cerevisiae* following exposure to UV radiation

8.2 Background Statement

Microbe: *Saccharomyces cerevisiae*

Species: Yeast

Type: Eukaryotic; Kingdom: Fungi

Yeast usually reproduces asexually by an asymmetric division process called budding. Under stressful condition, the diploid cells of yeast can pursue sporulation and haploid spores via meiosis.

Biochemical Engineering: A Laboratory Manual
Debabrata Das and Debayan Das
Copyright © 2021 Jenny Stanford Publishing Pte. Ltd.
ISBN 978-981-4877-36-7 (Hardcover), 978-1-003-11105-4 (eBook)
www.jennystanford.com

8.3 Theory

Microorganisms can be regarded as elementary biological particles able to undertake functional relationships with their surrounding environment. Although most microorganisms are beneficial and necessary for human beings, microbial activities may also have undesirable consequences. Therefore, it is essential to kill a wide variety of microorganisms to minimize their destructive effects.

The ability to destroy microorganisms is very important. It makes possible the aseptic technology techniques used in microbiological research, preservation of food, and treatment and prevention of disease.

Characteristically, the primary function of microbial interaction with the environment is the production of progeny. Hence, the single criterion of death of microorganism is the failure to reproduce in suitable environmental conditions. Physical and chemical agents affecting microbial activities to such an extent as to deprive microbial particles of the expected reproductive capability can be regarded as lethal agents. A wide range of physical and chemical lethal agents are available.

Heat ionizing and UV radiations are the most relevant physical lethal agents. Ultrasonic frequencies, pressure, surface tension, etc. are mostly employed as cell-disrupting agents in studying subcellular components. Chemical lethal agents consist of a wide range of components employed in the microbial inactivation process called disinfection. The most important disinfection compounds are H_2O_2, halogens, acids, alkalis, phenol, ethylene oxide, formaldehyde, glutaraldehyde, etc.

Most of the UV-C (the energy range that is most damaging to DNA) is filtered out of the sunlight by ozone. Normal cells repair most of the damage caused by UV-A and UV-B wavelengths that penetrate the atmosphere. Consequently, they are resistant to UV-B and UV-A in sunlight.

Most UV damage to DNA is in the form of pyrimidine dimers. Adjacent pyrimidine bases (thymine or cytosine) in one strand become joined by covalent bonds. A specific photo-reactivating enzyme (photolyase) uses energy from the visible light to split pyrimidine dimers. In other repair mechanisms, the enzyme removes the dimers and then patches the unaffected DNA.

Since most of the repair processes are so effective, only a source of high-energy UV-C (such as germicidal lamp) will produce substantial killing and mutation in normal yeast cells. A measurement of the dose of radiation absorbed by an organism is the rad, which is defined as 1 erg/g.

$$100 \, \text{rads} = 1 \, \text{Grey (Gy)}$$

Grey is the normally used unit for radiation exposure. Mutagenesis can occur from the effect of UV exposure providing structure like thymine dimers. When two adjacent thymines are exposed to UV light of wavelength 260 nm, they simultaneously fuse to form a dimer. The dimer thus formed no longer base-pairs with adenine and creates a noticeable kink, which will signal a base mismatch. If left to its own devices, DNA polymerase will "idle" at this site

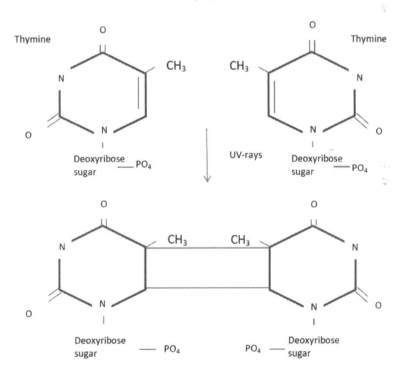

Figure 8.1 Formation of thymine dimer due to UV light.

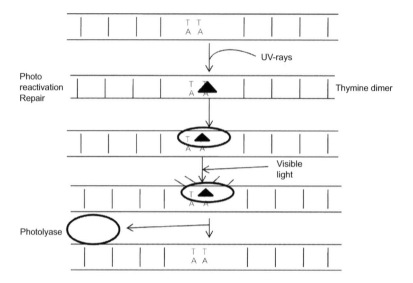

Figure 8.2 DNA repairing mechanism.

continuously converting dATP to dAMP because it gets caught in a loop of resource laying, then exciting the base in proofreading. DNA photolyases coded by phr genes allow bacteria to repair the damage to thymine dimers caused by UV exposure. The light energy is used by folate to transduce FADH to FADH$_2$. Electronically excited FADH$_2$ can transfer high energy to dimer causing the structure to break apart into separate thymine molecules.

The rate of destruction of the cell followed first-order kinetics as shown below:

$$-\frac{dx}{dt} = k_d\, x \tag{8.1}$$

$$-\int_{x_1}^{x_2} \frac{dx}{x} = k_d \int_{t_1}^{t_2} dt \tag{8.2}$$

$$\ln \frac{x_0}{x} = k_d(t_2 - t_1)$$

$$k_d = \frac{\ln \frac{x_1}{x_2}}{(t_2 - t_1)} \tag{8.3}$$

where k_d is the death rate constant (time^{-1}), x_1 is the initial viable cell concentration at time t_1, and x_2 is the initial viable cell concentration at time t_2 [1, 2].

8.4 Apparatus/Requirements

Apparatus: Laminar hood

Magnetic stirrer

Pipette

Stopwatch

Petri dishes

Test tubes

Chemicals

- 9.9 mL of 0.85% w/v NaCl solution: 6 test tubes
- 9 mL of 0.85% w/v NaCl solution: 12 test tubes
- 10 mL of 0.85% w/v NaCl solution: 2 test tubes

8.5 Media Composition

Working volume $= 200$ mL

Contents: Glucose $= 10$ g/L

Yeast extract $= 3$ g/L

Malt extract $= 3$ g/L

Peptone $= 5$ g/L

Agar $= 2\%$ w/v

8.6 Procedure

(1) In a Petri dish, 20 mL of yeast suspension (1 to 5×10^5 cells/mL, approximately) is taken.
(2) A sterile magnetic stirrer is added in the cell suspension.
(3) The UV lamp is kept about 5 cm above the Petri dish.
(4) The cover from the Petri dish is removed and irradiation is started.

(5) The sample is removed at 20 s interval, and it is continued up to 2 min.
(6) The serial dilution of the samples is made as per requirement.
(7) By using a sterile pipette, 0.1 mL of dilute sample is added in the Petri dishes containing solid medium.
(8) A viable count has to be carried out by staining with methylene blue using a hemocytometer.

8.7 Observation

Table 8.1 Viable cell concentration at different time exposure to UV rays

Time (s)	Dilution factor plated	Number of colonies	Number of viable cells/mL
0	10^4	810	81,000,000
20	10^4	104	10,400,000
40	10^4	42	4,200,000
60	10^2	480	4,801,000
80	10^2	30	30,000
100	10^2	60	6,000

Table 8.2 Calculated data

Time (s)	Number of variable cells/mL	x/x_0	$\ln(x/x_0)$
0	81,000,000	1	0
20	10,400,000	0.128395	−2.05264
40	4,200,000	0.051852	−2.95936
60	480,000	0.005926	−5.12842
80	30,000	0.00037	−7.90101
100	6,000	0.000074	−9.51044

Figure 8.3 is known as the kill curve. It is used for finding out the death rate constant of the cells upon UV exposure.

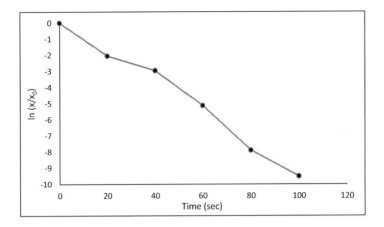

Figure 8.3 Destruction profile of viable yeast cells.

From Eq. 8.3,

$$k_d = \frac{\ln \frac{x_1}{x_2}}{(t_2 - t_1)}$$

Comparing with line equation

$$k_d = \text{slope} = 0.093 \text{ s}^{-1}$$

8.7.1 Sample Calculation

$$\text{Number of viable cells} = \frac{(\text{Number of colony}) \times (\text{Dilution factor})}{(\text{Volume of culture})}$$

At time t_1:

Number of colony $= 810$

Dilution factor $= 10^4$

Volume of culture $= 0.1$ mL

$$\text{Number of viable cells} = \frac{810 \times 10^4}{0.1} = 81,000,000/\text{mL} = x_0$$

At $t_2 = 60$ s:

Number of colony $= 480$

Dilution factor $= 10^2$

Volume of culture $= 100$ μL $= 0.1$ mL

Number of viable cells $= \dfrac{480 \times 10^2}{0.1} = 480,000/\text{mL} = x$

$$x/x_0 = \dfrac{81,000,000}{480,000} = 168.75$$

$$\ln(x/x_0) = \ln(168.75) = 5.13$$

Death constant $(k_d) = \dfrac{5.13}{60}\ \text{s}^{-1} = 0.0855\ \text{s}^{-1}$

8.8 Discussion

A microbial population is killed when exposed to a lethal agent. Cell death is generally logarithmic or exponential, i.e., the population will be reduced by the same fraction at constant intervals. Logarithm of the viable cell population number profiles gives a almost straight line plot. When the population has been greatly reduced, the rate of killing may slow due to the survival of a more resistant strain of microorganism.

Various factors influence the effectiveness of an UV sterilizer:

- **Size and type of microorganisms**: Larger organisms require a larger dose of UV radiation than smaller organisms.
- **Power of bulb**: The higher the wattage of UV bulb, the higher the dose of radiation.
- **UV penetration**: Higher water turbidity decreases the UV penetration. Salinity also affects penetration. The cleanliness of lamp or sleeve is important. If a film or mineral deposit covers the lamp, the light is partially or totally blocked. The distance of the lamp from the medium also influences the effectiveness of killing cells.
- **Contact time**: For a longer time of exposure, the contaminated substance is exposed to the UV light for a longer time. The killing population will be more.

- **Temperature**: UV light is best produced at temperatures of 104–110°F. A cooler temperature will result in less output.

8.9 Conclusion

UV rays are highly effective in killing *S. cerevisiae* than heat. The yeast cells die during exposure to UV rays mainly due to dimer formation between the two thymine molecules present in the DNA. This makes the DNA inactive.

References

1. Bailey, J. E. and Ollis, D. F., *Biochemical Engineering Fundamentals*, McGraw-Hill Inc., New Delhi, India, 2010.
2. Aiba, S., Humphrey, A. E., and Millis, N. F., *Biochemical Engineering*, Academic Press, 1973.

Experiment 9

Determination of Yeast Cell Density

Objective: To find out the density of *Saccharomyces cerevisiae*

9.1 Purpose

To determine the size and density of yeast cells using specific gravity bottles

9.2 Microorganism

Saccharomyces cerevisiae

Species: Yeast; Kingdom: Fungi

Natural ecology: Found primarily in ripe fruits

Optimum temperature: 30–35°C

Reproduction: Haploid cell → mitosis (building)

Diploid cells → Can either under mitosis or sporulation by entering meiosis

Biochemical Engineering: A Laboratory Manual
Debabrata Das and Debayan Das
Copyright © 2021 Jenny Stanford Publishing Pte. Ltd.
ISBN 978-981-4877-36-7 (Hardcover), 978-1-003-11105-4 (eBook)
www.jennystanford.com

9.3 Theory

Yeast forms one of the important subgroups of fungi. Although most fungi have relatively complex morphology, yeast is distinguished by its usual existence as single, small cells 5–30 μm long and 1–5 μm wide. But for experimental purpose, it is assumed that cell shapes are spherical. They usually show budding under the microscope.

Yeast can grow aerobically in MYG (malt extract, yeast extract, and glucose) medium. The cell suspension constitutes of both cells and media.

Let us assume m_y = mass of cells, m_c = mass of suspension, m_m = mass of media, V_y = volume of cell, V_c = volume of cell suspension, V_m = volume of media, ρ_y = density of cell, ρ_c = density of suspension, and ρ_m = density of media.

Now,

$$\text{Cell Suspension} = \text{Yeast cell} + \text{Media} \qquad (9.1)$$
$$(C) \qquad\qquad (Y) \qquad\quad (M)$$
$$m_c = m_y + m_m \qquad (9.2)$$
$$V_c = V_y + V_m \qquad (9.3)$$
$$\rho_c = \frac{m_c}{V_c}, \; \rho_y = \frac{m_y}{V_y}, \; \rho_c = \frac{m_m}{V_m} \qquad (9.4)$$

Let C be the volume fraction of cells in suspension.

$$C = \frac{\text{Volume of cells}}{\text{Volume of suspension}} = \frac{V_y}{V_c} \qquad (9.5)$$

But

$$\rho_y = \frac{m_y}{V_y}$$

Dividing the numerator and denominator by V_C, we get

$$\rho_y = \frac{m_y/V_c}{V_y/V_c} = \frac{\frac{(m_c - m_m)}{V_c}}{C} = \left(\frac{\frac{m_c}{V_c} - \frac{m_m}{V_c}}{C} \right)$$
$$= \frac{\left(\rho_c - \frac{m_m}{V_c} \right)}{C} = \frac{\left(\rho_c - \frac{m_m}{V_m} \times \frac{V_m}{V_c} \right)}{C} \qquad (9.6)$$
$$\rho_y = \frac{\left(\rho_c - \rho_m \frac{V_m}{V_c} \right)}{C} \qquad (9.7)$$

$$V_c = V_y + V_m \Rightarrow \frac{V_c}{V_c} = \frac{V_y}{V_c} + \frac{V_m}{V_c} \Rightarrow 1 = C + \frac{V_m}{V_c}$$

i.e., $\quad \dfrac{V_m}{V_c} = 1 - C$ $\hspace{4cm}$ (9.8)

Substituting in Eq. 9.7,

$$\rho_y = \frac{\rho_c - \rho_m(1 - C)}{C} \hspace{3cm} (9.9)$$

The above expression gives the density of yeast cells.

For visual counting of the number of cells, use a device called hemocytometer. It consists of a thick glass microscope slide with a regular indentation that creates a chamber. This chamber is engraved with a laser-etched grid of perpendicular lines. The device is carefully crafted so that the area bounded by the line and the depth of the chamber is known.

The microscope used in the experiment has an ocular micrometer fitted in its eye piece. This micrometer is a glass disk that has a ruled scale, which is used to measure the size of cells. The physical length of the marks depends on the degree of magnification.

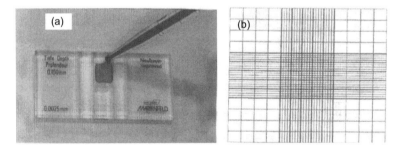

Figure 9.1   (a) Hemocytometer slide and (b) standard hemocytometer grid.

9.4 Requirements

- Specific gravity bottle
- Hemocytometer
- Ocular micrometer
- Microscope

- Slide and cover slips
- Centrifuge: Eppendorf centrifuge 5180R

Chemicals: KH_2PO_4 buffer (pH $= 5.0$)

Media:

Type: Complex media

Constituents: Glucose $= 10$ g/L; peptone $= 5$ g/L; yeast extract $= 3$ g/L; malt extract $= 3$ g/L; initial pH of medium $= 5.0$

9.5 Procedure

(1) An empty specific gravity bottle is weighed.
(2) For precise measurement of the volume of water, medium, etc., a specific gravity bottle of 10 mL is used.
(3) The weight of the bottle with water is taken.
(4) The weight of the bottle containing the medium is taken.
(5) The weight of the bottle with yeast cells suspended in buffer is also taken.
(6) To estimate the cell concentration, one drop of the cell suspension is taken and is put on the hemocytometer.
(7) The size of the cell is estimated with the help of an ocular micrometer fitted in the microscope. The ocular micrometer is calibrated with a stage micrometer at a particular magnification and the cell size is also measured at the same magnification.

9.6 Observation

To calibrate the ocular micrometer, a stage micrometer with known dimension is used. As observed under the microscope,

40 div of ocular scale $= 1$ div of stage scale

i.e., 40 div (ocular) $= 1$ div (stage)

Also 1 div (stage) $= 0.1$ mm $= 100$ μm

1 div (ocular) $= 100/40$ μm

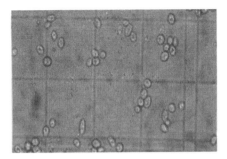

Figure 9.2   Morphology of the yeast cells (40× magnification).

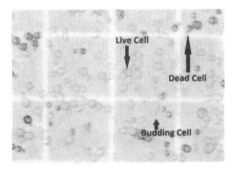

Figure 9.3   Difference between live and dead cells due to staining.

1 div (ocular) = 2.5 μm

Observed yeast cell size = 3 div (ocular)
$$= (3 \times 2.5)\ \mu m = 7.5\ \mu m$$

Thus, size of yeast cell = 7.5 μm.

From Eq. 9.9,

$$\rho_y = \frac{\rho_c - \rho_m\,(1 - C)}{C}$$

where ρ_y is the density of yeast cells, ρ_c is the density of suspension, ρ_m is the density of medium (broth), and C is the volume fraction of cell (C = Volume of cell/Volume of suspension).

$$\text{Number of cells} = \frac{(\text{Number of cells counted})}{\frac{(\text{Number of squares counted})}{(\text{Volume of one square of hemocytometer})}} \times \text{Dilution}$$

(Using hemocytometer)

According to specific gravity measurements,

$\rho_m = 1.009\,\text{g/cm}^3$

$\rho_c = 1.0079\,\text{g/cm}^3$

Size of yeast cell is 7.5 μm.

As observed under microscope,

Number of cells counted $= 174$

Number of squares counted $= 1$

Dilution $= 20$

$\therefore$ Number of cells $= 174 \times \dfrac{20}{0.0001} = 348 \times 10^5$ per mL

Total sample volume $= 10$ mL

$\therefore$ Total number of cells $= 343 \times 10^6$ cells

Assuming each cell to be spherical and similar in size,

Diameter of each cell $= 7.5$ μm

Radius of each cell $= 3.75$ μm

Volume of each cell $= \dfrac{4}{3}\pi r^3 = \dfrac{4}{3} \times \dfrac{22}{7} \times (3.75)^3$

$$= 220.98\ \mu\text{m}^3$$

$$= 220.98 \times 10^{-12}\ \text{cm}^3$$

Total volume of al cells $= 220.98 \times 10^{-12} \times 348 \times 10^6$

$$= 7.69 \times 10^{-2}\text{cm}^3$$

$$= 0.0769\ \text{cm}^3$$

$C = \dfrac{0.0769}{10} = 0.00769$

$\rho_y = \dfrac{1.009 - (1 - 0.00769) \times 1.0079}{0.00769}$

$\rho_y = 1.151\,\text{g/cm}^3 = 1.151\,\text{g/mL}$

9.7 Discussion

The hemocytometer gives the total cell count, both dead and viable. To distinguish between dead and viable cells, the sample is diluted with a particular stain, such as methylene blue. This staining method is also known as dye exclusion staining. It uses a diazo dye that selectively penetrates cell membranes of dead cells, coloring them, but is not absorbed by the membranes of live cells and the live cells are not stained (Fig. 9.3). When observed under a microscope, dead cells appear dark blue whereas live cells appear white.

Proper care should be taken while counting the numbers of cells. For large cells, we simply count the cells inside the four large corner squares and the middle one. For a dense suspension of small cells, we can count the cells in the four outer middle squares of the central squares or make a more dilute suspension. If a cell overlaps a ruling, count it as "in" if it overlaps the top or right ruling and "out" if it overlaps the bottom or left ruling. This is done to avoid counting the cells twice. Suspension should be dilute enough so that the cell or other particles do not overlap each other on the grid and be uniformly distributed.

The cover slip must be placed over the counting surface before the loading of sample (cell suspension). After addition, the sample is allowed to settle for a couple of minutes. Avoid moving the cover slips as it might introduce air bubbles and make counting difficult. The hemocytometer and coverslips are properly cleaned before use. Cover slips that are used for mounting on the hemocytometer are specially made to be thicker than the conventional microscope cover slips because they must be able to overcome the surface tension of a drop of liquid.

The advantage of using a hemocytometer is that it is quite cheap and fast. This makes them the preferred counting method in fast biological experiments in which it needs to be merely determined whether a cell culture has grown as expected. However, there are some limitations in using a hemocytometer:

- The culture examined needs to be diluted; else a high density of cells would lead to clumping, which would make counting difficult. This is always a factor of inaccuracy due to dilution.

- If the suspension is too dilute, the sample size will not be enough to make a strong influence about the concentration in the original mixture.

Accurate calculation of cell size and density has many applications such as cell processing for downstream analysis. Accurate cell counts are needed for many tests such as PCR and flow cytometry, while some require high cell viability and also tracking the growth profile of any cell/microbe [1–3].

9.8 Conclusion

The density of the wet yeast cell (*S. cerevisiae*) in the present study is found to be 1.151 g/mL, which is closer to the reported value of 1.112 g/mL. Little difference in yeast cell density may be due to the presence of some insoluble particles.

References

1. Bailey, J. E. and Ollis, D. F., *Biochemical Engineering Fundamentals*, McGraw-Hill Inc., New Delhi, India, 2010.
2. Shuler, M. L. and Kargi, F., *Bioprocess Engineering: Basic Concepts*, Second Edition, Prentice-Hall Inc., New Delhi, India, 2002.
3. Doran, P. M., *Bioprocess Engineering Principles*, Second Edition, Academic Press, Waltham, USA, 2012.

Experiment 10

Biohydrogen Production in Batch Process

Objective: Determination of the kinetic constants of mixed acido-genic bacterial culture for biohydrogen production

10.1 Purpose

To study biohydrogen production in a batch process in a customized bioreactor and to measure

- Maximum specific growth rate μ_{max}
- Saturation constant K_S
- True growth yield coefficient $Y'_{x/s}$
- Maintenance coefficient m
- Cumulative hydrogen production P
- Specific hydrogen production rate $\dfrac{1}{x}\dfrac{dp}{dt}$
- Product yield coefficient $Y_{p/s}$
- Luedeking and Piret constants α and β

Biochemical Engineering: A Laboratory Manual
Debabrata Das and Debayan Das
Copyright © 2021 Jenny Stanford Publishing Pte. Ltd.
ISBN 978-981-4877-36-7 (Hardcover), 978-1-003-11105-4 (eBook)
www.jennystanford.com

10.2 Theory

Environmental pollution due to the use of fossil fuels as well as their shortfall makes it necessary to find alternative energy sources that are environmentally friendly and renewable. Hydrogen satisfies these requirements because when it burns, it produces only water. There are various processes for biohydrogen production: dark fermentation, photo-fermentation, biophotolysis, and hybrid fermentation. However, fermentative (dark) hydrogen production is more feasible and widely used. During dark fermentation, the substrate is degraded to cell mass, hydrogen, carbon dioxide, and soluble metabolites.

Biohydrogen can be produced by different raw materials such as glucose, sugarcane molasses, and starchy materials.

The stoichiometry of hydrogen production from glucose by the acetate pathway is as follows:

$$C_6H_{12}O_6 + 2H_2O \rightarrow 2CH_3COOH + 2CO_2 + 4H_2 \qquad (10.1)$$

Theoretically, 1 mol of glucose produces 4 mol of hydrogen. Biohydrogen is produced by the fermentation of glucose under anaerobic condition. Hydrogenase is the principal enzyme that catalyzes the conversion of protons to hydrogen.

Hydrogen can also be produced by the butyrate pathway wherein 2 mol of hydrogen is produced from 1 mol of glucose. During hydrogen production, there exists some relationship among various parameters such as substrate consumption, rate of cell growth, and rate of hydrogen production.

The Luedeking–Piret model can be used to find out the product formation:

$$\frac{dp}{dt} = \alpha \frac{dx}{dt} + \beta x \qquad (10.2)$$

where p is the product concentration (g/L), α is the growth-associated coefficient, β is the nongrowth-associated coefficient (h^{-1}), x is the cell mass concentration (g/L), and t is time (h).

$$\frac{1}{x}\frac{dp}{dt} = \frac{\alpha}{x}\frac{dx}{dt} + \beta \qquad (10.3)$$

$$\vartheta = \alpha\mu + \beta \qquad (10.4)$$

where ϑ is the specific product formation rate (h^{-1}).

10.3 Materials Required

Microorganism: Acidogenic mixed consortium

Experimental setup comprises the following:

- 500 mL working volume customized bioreactors
- Trap, CO_2 absorber, gas collectors, pipettes
- Gas chromatograms
- Nephloturbidometer
- Spectrophotometer
- Centrifuge
- Dinitrosalicyclic (DNS) acid solution
- Test tubes

10.4 Medium

The constituents of the medium are

- Glucose $= 10$ g/L
- Malt extract $= 10.0$ g/L
- Yeast extract $= 4.0$ g/L
- pH $= 6.5$
- Temperature $= 37°$C

10.5 Procedure

(1) The experimental setup is assembled.
(2) The bioreactor having a working volume of 500 mL is inoculated with 50% v/v seed culture grown overnight.
(3) The temperature of the experimental setup is maintained at $37°$C by a circulating water bath.
(4) The reactor is sparged with nitrogen gas (99.9% pure) to maintain anaerobicity.

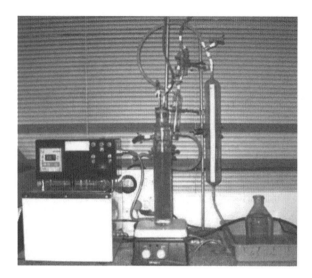

Figure 10.1 Experimental setup for biohydrogen production in a batch process.

(5) For the selective absorption of CO_2 produced during the reaction, 40% w/v KOH solution is used.

(6) The remaining gas (containing mostly H_2) is collected in a gas collector by the displacement of 10% w/v saline water at normal temperature and atmospheric pressure.

(7) For analysis, 5 mL of fermentation broth is drawn at an hourly interval maintaining aseptic condition. This is used to analyze the biomass and glucose concentration.

10.6 Discussion

From Fig. 10.5, from the intercept, $\mu_{max} = \dfrac{1}{1.7965} = 0.556\,h^{-1}$

Minimum doubling time, $t_{d\,(minimum)} = 1.25\,h$.

From the slope, $\dfrac{K_S}{\mu_{max}} = 19.837$

$K_S = 19.837 \times 0.556 = 11.04\,g/L$

Table 10.1 Experimental and calculated data of biohydrogen production process

Time (h)	H_2 (mL)	H_2 (mL/L)	S (g/L)	x (g/L)	1/x (L/g)	$\frac{dx}{dt}$ (g/L h)	$\mu = \frac{1}{x}\frac{dx}{dt}$ (h^{-1})
0	0	0	15.00	0.18	5.56	—	—
1	27.3	54.6	14.30	0.28	3.57	0.12	0.41
2	54.6	109.2	14.10	0.41	2.44	0.13	0.30
3	95.6	191.1	13.10	0.53	1.89	0.10	0.19
4	177.5	354.9	12.90	0.61	1.64	0.19	0.30
5	300.3	600.6	8.95	0.90	1.11	0.32	0.36
6	363.6	7.7.1	6.75	1.25	0.30	0.23	0.22
7	423.2	846.3	5.50	1.45	0.69	0.32	0.22
8	498.2	996.5	4.50	1.33	0.53	0.27	0.14
9	577.4	1154.3	4.15	1.99	0.50	0.12	0.06
10	641.6	1233.1	3.50	2.12	0.47	−0.01	0
11	686.6	1373.2	3.92	1.98	0.51	−0.07	−0.03
12	718.0	1436.0	3.90	1.99	0.50	−0.04	−0.02
13	718	1436.0	3.39	1.90	0.53	−1.00	−0.52

Table 10.2 Calculated data for the determination of product formation kinetics

Time (h)	$\frac{dx}{dt}$ (g/L h)	$\frac{ds}{dt}$ (g/L h)	$\frac{dp}{dt}$ (mL/L h)	$Y_{x/s}$	$Y_{p/x}$ (mL/g)	$Y_{p/x}$ (ml/g)	μh^{-1}	$\vartheta = \frac{1}{x}\frac{dp}{dt}$ (mL/g h)
1	0.12	0.45	54.6	0.256	474.78	121.3	0.41	195
2	0.13	0.85	68.25	0.147	546	80.29	0.305	166.46
3	0.1	0.60	122.35	0.167	1223.5	204.75	0.19	231.7925
4	0.19	2.075	204.75	0.089	1106.56	93.67	0.30	335.66
5	0.32	3.075	191.10	0.104	597.19	62.15	0.36	212.3
6	0.28	1.725	122.85	0.159	446.73	71.22	0.22	98.23
7	0.32	1.125	129.7	0.28	411.75	115.29	0.217	89.45
8	0.27	0.675	154.25	0.4	571.296	236.51	0.14	82.05
9	0.12	0.50	143.26	0.24	1193.79	949.57	0.06	71.99

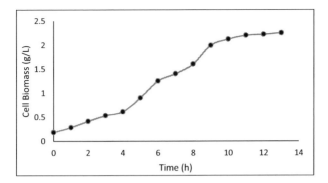

Figure 10.2   Cell mass concentration profile.

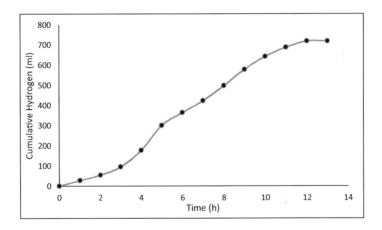

Figure 10.3   Cumulative hydrogen production profile.

Again from Fig. 10.6, from the intercept, $\beta = 48.73$ (mL/g h)

From the slope, $\alpha = 474.28 \left(\dfrac{\text{mL}}{\text{g}} \right)$

From experimental data, it has been observed that the cell mass concentration gradually increases with progress in time. Similarly, the product (hydrogen) formation increases with time. The substrate concentration decreases very slowly in the first 4 h and then gradually decreases over time. The substrate concentration is nearly constant in the last 4 h of the experiment.

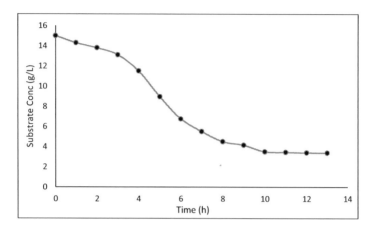

Figure 10.4 Substrate concentration profile.

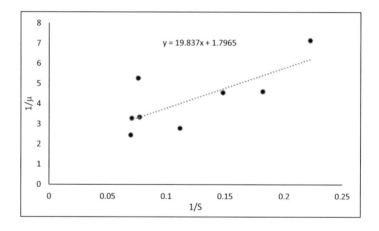

Figure 10.5 Plot of $1/\mu$ versus $1/S$.

Hydrogen production through dark fermentation has many advantages in comparison to other biological hydrogen production methods because of its ability to produce hydrogen from renewable resources such as carbohydrate-rich wastes, with the minimum external input of energy. It has been reported that an acidogenic mixed culture has similar hydrogen production ability like pure culture such as *Enterobacter cloacae*.

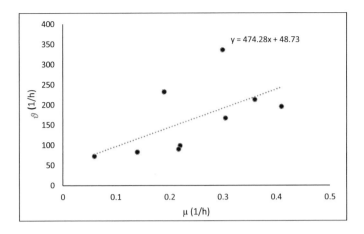

Figure 10.6 Plot of ϑ versus μ.

From the experimental data, we observe that the α value is much higher than the β value. So it can be assumed that hydrogen production may be considered a growth-associated product.

The bacterial species metabolize simple sugars using the glycolytic pathway where they are converted to pyruvate. It is then oxidized by the enzyme pyruvate ferredoxin oxidoreductase to yield acetyl CoA, CO_2, and reduced ferredoxin. Reoxidation of the reduced ferredoxin is catalyzed by the enzyme hydrogenase and generates hydrogen gas.

However, dark fermentation is reported to produce low H_2 yield. Various pretreatment methods claim to produce better results. Pretreatment of substrates such as algal biomass and water hyacinth helps to accelerate the hydrolysis step. This reduces the impact of the rate-limiting step and augments the anaerobic digestion to enhance H_2 generation. Several pretreatment procedures such as heat shock, chemical agents, acid shock, and alkali shock are employed on a variety of mixed culture for the selective enrichment of acidogenic H_2 producing inoculum. The pH plays a critical role in governing the metabolic pathways of the organism where the activity of the acidogenic group of bacteria is considered to be crucial.

Facultative H_2-producing anaerobes face no problem when exposed to oxygen. However, obligate anaerobe methanogens die.

Lower H_2-production rate is reported when oxygen stress is applied to the system. It has also been reported that an acidic pH close to 6.5 can increase the ability of hydrogen-producing bacteria, thereby improving the yield [1–6].

10.7 Conclusion

Mixed acidogenic bacterial culture is found suitable for hydrogen production. The minimum doubling time of the culture is 1.25 h, which is much smaller than that of *E. cloacae* IIT-BT 08 grown under aerobic condition. The cell growth rate of the aerobic culture is higher than that of the anaerobically grown culture.

References

1. Das, D., Khanna, N., and Nag Dasgupta, C., *Biohydrogen Production: Fundamentals and Technology Advances*, CRC Press, 2014.
2. Kumari, S. and Das, D., Improvement of biohydrogen production using acidogenic culture, *International Journal of Hydrogen Energy*, **42**: 4083–4094, 2017.
3. Nath, K. and Das, D., Modeling and optimization of fermentative hydrogen production, *Bioresource Technology*, **102**: 8569–8581, 2011.
4. Balachandar, G., Varanasi Jhansi, L., Singh, V., Singh, H., and Das, D., Biological hydrogen production via dark fermentation: A holistic approach from lab-scale to pilot-scale, *International Journal of Hydrogen Energy*, **45**: 5202–5215, 2020.
5. Das, D. and Nejat Veziroglu, T., Hydrogen production by biological processes: A survey of literature, *International Journal of Hydrogen Energy*, **26**: 13–28, 2001.
6. Kumar, N. and Das, D., Enhancement of hydrogen production by *Enterobacter cloacae* IIT-BT 08, *Process Biochemistry*, **35**: 589–594, 2000 (Erratum 35; 9: 1074).

Experiment 11

Continuous Biohydrogen Production in a Chemostat

Objective: To study the kinetics of the continuous biohydrogen production process using *Enterobacter cloacae* IIT-BT 08

11.1 Purpose

Determination of the kinetic constants of *E. cloacae* in the continuous biohydrogen production process

11.2 Theory

Hydrogen as a fuel provides an advantageous option in comparison to fossil fuels due to the increasing environmental pollution. H_2 can be used for the generation of electricity by fuel cells, and on combustion it only produces H_2O. This is in contrary to CO_2 produced by fossil fuels, which has greenhouse effect. In addition, hydrogen is a better fuel as it has the highest calorific value. It can be produced from organic wastes using the dark fermentation process. Since it is free from SO_2, it can be directly used in fuel cells.

Biochemical Engineering: A Laboratory Manual
Debabrata Das and Debayan Das
Copyright © 2021 Jenny Stanford Publishing Pte. Ltd.
ISBN 978-981-4877-36-7 (Hardcover), 978-1-003-11105-4 (eBook)
www.jennystanford.com

In a continuous stirred tank reactor (also known as a chemostat), one can carry out the process of H_2 production (Fig. 11.1). This process has advantages in comparison to a batch culture, since the microbial growth here can be kept in a desired log phase where maximum hydrogen production can be achieved since hydrogen production is a growth-associated product. The reactor is initially operated in the batch mode. The continuous mode of operation is started when the rate of hydrogen production is maximum. At a particular flow rate, steady-state condition can be achieved after infinite time when the concentration of different components present in the fermentation broth remains constant. A completely sterile medium ($x_0 = 0$) is fed to the chemostat. The cell growth rate depends on the dilution rate.

$$\text{Dilution rate} D = \frac{F}{V} (\text{time}^{-1}) \tag{11.1}$$

where F is the volumetric flow rate of the medium (vol/time), and V is the working or liquid volume in the reactor.

Hydraulic retention time (HRT): It is also known as the average length of time the medium remains in the reactor. It is considered the reaction time.

$$HRT = \theta = \frac{V}{F} = \frac{1}{D} \tag{11.2}$$

The cell mass balance in the chemostat may expressed as

Rate of cell mass input + Rate of cell mass formation = Rate of cell mass output + Rate of death of cell mass + Rate of accumulation of cell mass

$$F x_0 + r_x V = F x + r_d V + \frac{d(xV)}{dt} \tag{11.3}$$

where r_x is the rate of cell mass formation, x_0 is the inflow cell mass concentration, x is the outflow cell mass concentration, r_d is the rate of death of cell mass, and t is time.

Under steady-state condition, the rate of cell mass accumulation is $\frac{d(xV)}{dt} = 0$.

Assuming $x_0 = 0$ and $r_d = 0$, Eq. 11.3 may be written as follows:

$$r_x V = F x \tag{11.4}$$

$$\frac{1}{x} r_x = \frac{F}{V}$$

$$\mu = \frac{F}{V} = D \tag{11.5}$$

Substrate balance in the chemostat may be written as

$$F S_0 + 0 = F S + (-rs) V + \frac{d (V S)}{dt} \qquad (11.6)$$

At steady state, accumulation, $\dfrac{d (V S)}{dt} = 0$

Again, $-r_s = -\dfrac{ds}{dt} = \dfrac{1}{Y_x/s} \dfrac{dx}{dt} = \dfrac{1}{Y_{x/s}} \mu x$

Equation 11.6 may be written as

$$F S_0 = F S + (-r_s) V$$

$$F S_0 = F S + \frac{\mu x V}{Y_{x/s}} \qquad (11.7)$$

$$\left(\frac{F}{V} \right) s_0 = \left(\frac{F}{V} \right) S + \left(\frac{1}{Y_{x/s}} \frac{dx}{dt} \right), \text{ since } \tfrac{dx}{dt} = \mu x$$

$$D (S_0 - S) = \frac{1}{Y_{x/s}} \mu x \qquad (11.8)$$

Again, under steady-state condition and sterile feed,

$$\mu = D = \frac{\mu_{\max} S}{K_s + S} \qquad (11.9)$$

So steady-state substrate concentration is

$$S = \frac{D k_s}{\mu_{\max} - D} \qquad (11.10)$$

Again,

$$Y_{x/s} = \frac{x - x_0}{S_0 - S} = \frac{x}{S_0 - S}$$

where in the case of sterile feed, $x_0 = 0$

$$\Rightarrow X = Y_{x/s} \left(S_0 - \frac{D K_s}{\mu_{\max} - D} \right) \qquad (11.11)$$

Cell mass productivity

$$(r_x) = \frac{\text{Cell mass produced}}{\text{Time}} = DX \qquad (11.12)$$

$$r_x = Y_{x/s} \left(D S_0 - \frac{D^2 K_s}{\mu_{\max} - D} \right) \qquad (11.13)$$

At steady-state condition, $\dfrac{d\,(DX)}{dD} = 0$, D_{max} is obtained.

Since $D_{max} < \mu_{max}$

$$D_{max} = \mu_{max}\left(1 - \sqrt{\dfrac{K_S}{K_S + S_0}}\right) \qquad (11.14)$$

Operation of the chemostat at D_{max} gives the maximum rate of cell mass production from the reactor.

$$\text{At } D = D_{max},$$

Maximum cell mass productivities,

$$Q_{x(max)} = x\,D_{max}$$

$$= Y_{x/s}\left(S_0 D_{max} - \dfrac{D_{max}^2 K_S}{\mu_{max} - D_{max}}\right) \qquad (11.15)$$

The washout of the cell mass will take place at a high dilution rate where "x" reduces to zero. This dilution rate is termed $D_{washout}$. It is the situation when the cell mass growth rate can no longer keep up with this dilution rate. As the dilution rate (D) increases, the steady-state substrate concentration (S) increases slowly at first, then more rapidly to S_0 as D reaches $D_{washout}$. Correspondingly, the steady-state cell mass concentration decreases to zero. So $D_{washout}$ may written as

$$D_{washout} = \dfrac{\mu_{max} S_0}{K_S + S_0} \qquad (11.16)$$

$$D_{max} < D_{washout} \leq \mu_{max}$$

From Eq. 11.9, $D = \dfrac{\mu_{max} S}{K_S + S}$

$$\dfrac{1}{D} = \dfrac{K_S}{\mu_{max}}\dfrac{1}{S} + \dfrac{1}{\mu_{max}} \qquad (11.17)$$

The values of K_S and μ_{max} can be obtained from the plot $1/D$ versus $1/S$. The slope is equal to $\dfrac{K_S}{\mu_{max}}$, and the intercept gives the values of $\dfrac{1}{\mu_{max}}$.

The chemostat works best at lower dilution rates when the changes in x and S are small. It may not be practical to operate at D_{max}, which is close to $D_{washout}$. This is because a small variation in the dilution rate in this region causes a large fluctuation in x and

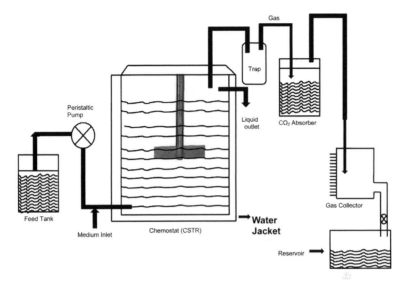

Figure 11.1 Schematic diagram of a chemostat.

S. However, the washout problem can be overcome by (a) recycling the cell mass and (b) using immobilized whole cell. To keep the cell concentration higher than the normal steady-state level, cell mass in the effluent can be recycled back to the reactor to operate the system at a higher dilution rate.

In the present experimental study, *Enterobacter cloacae* IIT-BT 08 is used to produce H_2 in a chemostat (CSTR). It is a facultative anaerobe, which produces H_2 in anaerobic conditions.

11.3 Materials

The following materials are required: bioreactor (jacketed), trap, CO_2 absorber, gas collector, peristaltic pumps, pipettes, gas chromatograph, spectrophotometer, centrifuge, DNS solution, test tubes.

Medium: Dextrose (10 g/L), malt extract (10 g/L), yeast extract (4 g/L), pH $= 6.5$

11.4 Procedure

The continuous H_2 production is carried out in a 500 mL glass double-jacketed reactor. The temperature of the reactor is maintained at 37°C by using a temperature-controlled circulating water bath. Anaerobic condition in the reactor is maintained by sparging N_2 gas for a fixed period. The system is initially operated in the batch mode and is shifted to the continuous mode when the rate of H_2 production reaches its peak. During the continuous process, the sterile feed is operated at different dilution rates (0.1, 0.15, 0.2, 0.25 h^{-1}). The feeding was done with the help of the peristaltic pump (PP). In the pump, the fluid is contained within a flexible tube (e.g., silicone tube) fitted inside the pump casing. The actual pumping principle, called peristalsis, is based on alternating compression and relaxation of the hose or tube, drawing content in and propelling product away from the pump. Samples from the reactor are withdrawn at regular intervals for the estimation of reducing sugar and cell mass concentration. The gas mixture was allowed to pass through 40% w/v KOH solution for the absorption of CO_2. The filled gas was collected in a graduated water-displacement system at ambient temperature and pressure.

11.5 Observation

Experimental results and the calculated data are shown in Tables 11.1 and 11.2. Different plots on the basis of the experimental data are shown in Figs. 11.2–11.4.

Table 11.1 Cumulative hydrogen production in the batch process

Time (h)	Cumulative hydrogen production (mL/L)
0	0
1	60
2	150
3	320
4	490
5	700
6	820

Table 11.2 Analysis of substrate and products of the chemostat at different dilution rates

Dilution rate (D) (h^{-1})	Rate of hydrogen production (mL/Lh)	Steady-state substrate (S) (g/L)	Substrate conversion efficiency (%)	Steady-state cell concentration (x) (g/L)
0.1	100	1.34	86.6	2.45
0.15	120	2.8	72	2.28
0.2	165	4.2	58	2.05
0.25	230	6.7	33	1.92

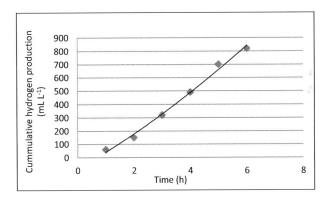

Figure 11.2 Cumulative hydrogen production profile in the batch process.

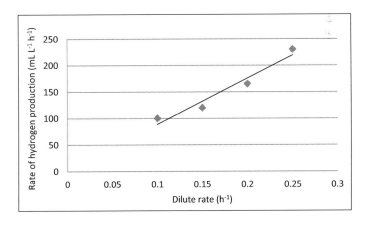

Figure 11.3 Steady-state hydrogen production at different dilution rates.

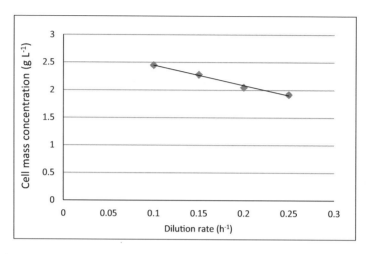

Figure 11.4   Steady-state cell mass concentration at different dilution rates.

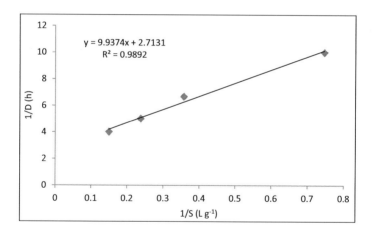

Figure 11.5   Plot of $1/D$ versus $1/S$.

From Fig. 11.5, intercept $= \dfrac{1}{\mu_{\text{max}}} = 2.713$

Therefore, $\mu_{\text{max}} = 0.37 \text{ h}^{-1}$

Slope $= \dfrac{K_s}{\mu_{\text{max}}} = 9.937$

Therefore, $K_s = 3.67 \text{ g/L}$

From Eq. 11.15,

$$D_{max} = \mu_{max}\left(1 - \sqrt{\frac{K_s}{K_s + S_0}}\right) = 0.37\left(1 - \sqrt{\frac{3.67}{3.67 + 10}}\right) = 0.18\,h^{-1}$$

From Eq. 11.17,

$$D_{washout} = \frac{\mu_{max}S_0}{K_s + S_0} = \frac{0.37 \times 10}{3.67 + 10} = 0.27\,h^{-1}$$

11.6 Discussion

A chemostat has certain advantages over the batch process. One can run the process at a particular phase of growth for an infinite time. One can also check the effect different components present in the medium on the cell growth kinetics. It has greater productivity in comparison to a batch process. A disadvantage is that this process is not suitable to study the life cycle of a cell. However, we need to run a batch process to determine the life cycle of an organism.

The downtime in a batch process is the major drawback. There is no downtime in a chemostat. Downtime is considered an idle time of the reactor when no reaction takes place. In a chemostat under steady-state condition, the solid retention time (SRT) (or mean cell residence time) becomes equal to HRT. However, SRT >HRT in the case of a chemostat with cell mass recycling.

With increase in the dilution rate, the rate of H_2 production increases. On further increase in the dilution rate, the washout situation might occur. To avoid washout, one can use cell recycling, immobilization, etc. The results are close to that reported in the literature due to minimum experimental errors (Das, Khanna, and Nag Dasgupta, 2014).

11.7 Conclusion

Enterobacter cloacae IIT-BT 08 is reported to produce hydrogen at a faster rate under anaerobic condition. The maximum rate of hydrogen production after 9 h of fermentation is 143 mL/L h in a batch process. However, in continuous fermentation, the rate of hydrogen production is 230 mL/L h, which is much higher than that in the batch process. This indicates that the continuous process is suitable for biohydrogen production.

References

1. Das, D., Khanna, N., and Nag Dasgupta, C., *Biohydrogen Production: Fundamentals and Technology Advances*, CRC Press, 2014.
2. Kumar, N. and Das, D., Continuous hydrogen production by immobilized Enterobacter cloacae IIT-BT 08 using lignocellulosic materials as solid matrices, *Enzyme and Microbial Technology*, **29**(4–5): 280–287, 2001.
3. Kumar, N. and Das, D., Enhancement of hydrogen production by Enterobacter cloacae IIT-BT 08, *Process Biochemistry*, **35**(6): 589–594, 2000 (Erratum 35; 9: 1074).

Experiment 12

Electricity Generation by Microbial Fuel Cells

Objective: Electricity generation from organic wastes using microbial fuel cells

12.1 Purpose

To study bioelectricity generation with simultaneous wastewater treatment in a batch culture and to determine

- Current density
- Power density
- Columbic efficiency

12.2 Microorganism

Microorganism: *Halomonas* sp.

Type: Facultative anaerobe

Specialty: Exoelectrogens

Exoelectrogens refer to the microorganisms that can transfer electrons extracellularly. Electrons undergoing exocytosis in this

Biochemical Engineering: A Laboratory Manual
Debabrata Das and Debayan Das
Copyright © 2021 Jenny Stanford Publishing Pte. Ltd.
ISBN 978-981-4877-36-7 (Hardcover), 978-1-003-11105-4 (eBook)
www.jennystanford.com

fashion are produced following ATP production using an electron transport chain during oxidative phosphorylation. The final electron acceptor of an exoelectrogen is found extracellularly and can be a strong oxidizing agent in an aqueous solution or a solid conductor/electron acceptor.

12.3 Theory

Microbial fuel cells (MFCs) are electrochemical transducers that drive current by using bacteria and mimicking bacterial interactions found in nature. In a broader sense, MFCs are a bioelectrochemical system capable of directly transforming chemical energy into electrical energy using exoelectrogen or electrogenic bacteria. A prototype MFC typically consists of anode and cathode chambers. They are physically separated by a proton exchange membrane (PEM) (Fig. 12.1). Microbes oxidize biodegradable organic substrate and produce electron at the anode. Electrons are produced by the conductive materials containing a resistor or operated under a load.

In the cathode chamber, protons react with oxygen in the presence of equivalent electrons to form water. One MFC can produce 1.1 V theoretically as open-circuit potential (OCP) where anodic (while acetate is utilized as substrate) and cathodic half-cell potentials are 0.3 V and 0.805 V, respectively. However, the range 0.55–0.8 V is reported as OCP due to the high internal resistance of MFC.

The organic matter present in the wastewater is used by the microorganism. Microbes utilize the wastewater as their nutrient source and electron source for carrying out their metabolic process. In this process, they degrade the organic matter. Hence, an MFC performs two tasks: producing electricity and wastewater treatment.

12.3.1 Reactions Taking Place at the Anode

$$CH_3COO^- + 4H_2O \xrightarrow[\text{oxidation}]{\text{Microbial}} 2HCO_3^- + 9H^+ + 8e^- \qquad (12.1)$$

Anodic half-cell potential can be calculated by Eq. 12.2.

$$E_{An} = E_{An}^\circ - \frac{RT}{8F} \ln \frac{[CH_3COO^-]}{[HCO_3^-]^2 [H^+]^9} \qquad (12.2)$$

Assuming $E_{An}^\circ = 0.187\,V$, $[CH_3COO^-] = 5\,mM$, $[HCO_3^-] = 5\,mM$,

temperature $= 25°C$, we get

$$E_{An} = 0.187 - \frac{(8.314 \times 298)}{3 \times (9.65 \times 10^4)} \ln \frac{0.005}{(0.005)^2(10^{-7})^9}$$

$$E_{An} = -0.2998\,V \qquad (12.3)$$

12.3.2 Reactions Taking Place at the Cathode

$$\frac{1}{2}O_2 + 2H^+ + 2e^- \xrightarrow{\text{Reduction}} H_2O \qquad (12.4)$$

Cathodic half-cell potential can be calculated by Eq. 12.5.

$$E_{cat} = E_{cat}^\circ - \frac{RT}{4F} \ln \frac{1}{[o_2][H^+]^4} \qquad (12.5)$$

Assuming

$$E_{cat}^\circ = 1.229\,V \text{ at pH} = 7$$

$$E_{cat} = 1.229 - \frac{(8.314 \times 298)}{4 \times (9.65 \times 10^4)} \ln \frac{1}{(0.2)\left(10^{-7}\right)^4}$$

$$E_{cat} = 0.805\,V \qquad (12.6)$$

$$E_{tot} = E_{cat} - E_{An} = (0.805 + 0.298)\,V$$

$$E_{tot} = 1.103\,V = \text{Total open-circuit voltage} \qquad (12.7)$$

We know that

$$P = I \times V$$

where P is power (W), I is current (A), and V is voltage (V).

Again

$$\text{Current density, } I_d = \frac{V}{R\,A_{anode}} I_d\,(A/cm^2) \qquad (12.8)$$

where R is the external resistance (Ω), A_{anode} is the projected surface of anode (cm^2).

$$\text{Coulombic efficiency, } C_E = \frac{8It_b}{FV_{AN}\Delta C} C_E \qquad (12.9)$$

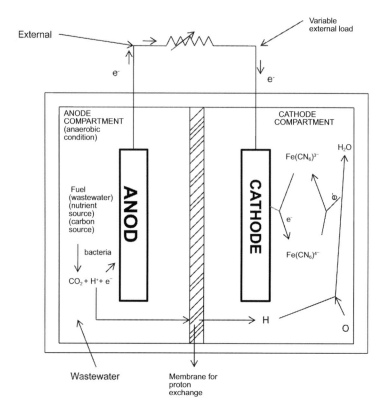

Figure 12.1   Schematic diagram of a microbial fuel cell.

where F is the Faraday constant (96,485 C/mol), I is the current generation at a particular external resistance (close circuit), ΔC = removed chemical oxygen demand (COD) (g/L), V_{AN} is the working volume of anode (L), and t_b is the batch time (s).

MFC in the open-circuit mode, $V = 0.75$ V.

12.4 Materials

Double-chambered MFC reactor, digital multimeter, data acquisition system, Ag/AgCl–KCl (+197 mV) reference electrode, resistance box, test tubes, pH meter.

COD digester (HACH DRB 200)

Spectrophotometer: HACH DRB 2800

12.4.1 Medium

Synthetic acetate-based wastewater (initial COD = 3000 mg/L)

$$CH_3COONa = \frac{3.843\,g}{L}, \; CaCl_2 \cdot 2H_2O = 0.75\,g/L$$

$$NaHCO_3 = 4.5\,g/L, \; MgSO_4 \cdot 7H_2O = 0.06\,g/L$$

$$NH_4Cl = 0.954\,g/L, \; FeSO_4 \cdot 7H_2O = 10\,mg/L$$

$$K_2HPO_4 = 0.081\,g/L, \; NiSO_4 \cdot 6H_2O = 0.526\,mg/L$$

$$kH_2PO_4 = 0.27\,g/L, \; MnSO_4 \cdot H_2O = 0.526\,mg/L$$

$$H_3BO_3 = 0.106\,mg/L, \; ZnSO_4 \cdot 7H_2O = 0.106\,mg/L$$

$$CoCl_2 \cdot 6H_2O = 52.6\,\mu g/L, CuSO_4 \cdot 5H_2O = 4.5\,\mu g/L$$

$$(NH_4)_6\,Mo_7O_{24} \cdot 4H_2O = 52.6\,\mu g/L$$

$$pH = 7.0$$

12.5 Procedure

12.5.1 Polarization

(1) The batch is run for at least 36 h employing 10% V/V pretreated consortia grown overnight (Figs. 12.2–12.4).
(2) The reactor is sparged with nitrogen gas (99.9% pure) to maintain anaerobicity.
(3) Once voltage generation in the closed-circuit mode reaches a steady state, polarization curves can be obtained by varying the external resistance box (range: 90,000 Ω to 1 Ω) in a stepwise manner and the voltage drop in each step is measured using a multimeter.
(4) The average time required to take stable readings is about 3–7 min. After taking a closed-circuit reading, the circuit is opened and is again closed to take fresh readings.

(5) From the anode chamber, 5 mL of the broth is drawn after the completion of batch process for analysis of COD removal and calculation of Columbic efficiency.

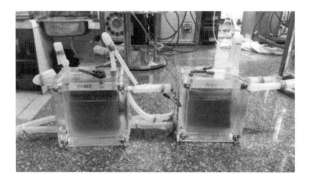

Figure 12.2   Experimental setup of microbial fuel cell before inoculation.

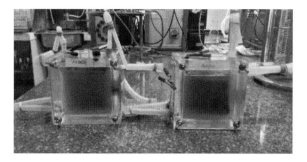

Figure 12.3   Experimental setup of microbial fuel cell after inoculation.

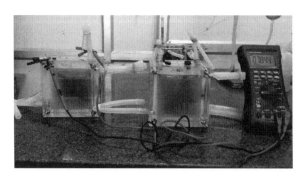

Figure 12.4   Experimental setup of microbial fuel cell after 36 h incubation.

12.6 Observation

12.6.1 Data for Polarization Study

$V_{An} = 400$ mL $= 400 \times 10^{-6}$ m^3, working volume (V_R)

$$= 275 \text{ mL} = 275 \times 10^{-6} \text{ m}^3$$

Surface area of anode $(A_{An}) = \dfrac{8}{2} \times \dfrac{8}{2} = \dfrac{64 \text{ cm}^2}{4}$

$$= 16 \text{ cm}^2 = 16 \times 10^{-4} \text{ m}^2$$

Experimental data of MFC is shown in Table 12.1. Polarization and power density curves are depicted in Fig. 12.5.

Table 12.1 Data on the performance of the MFC using different loads (external resistance)

External resistance (Ω)	Voltage (V)	Current (A)	Power (W)	Current density (A/m³)	Power density (W/m³)
90000	0.70600	7.84E-06	5.54E-06	0.02853	0.02014
80000	0.70600	8.83E-06	6.23E-06	0.03209	0.02266
70000	0.70600	1.01E-05	7.12E-06	0.03668	0.02589
60000	0.70600	1.18E-05	8.31E-06	0.04279	0.03021
50000	0.70600	1.41E-05	9.97E-06	0.05135	0.03625
40000	0.70600	1.77E-05	1.25E-05	0.06418	0.04531
30000	0.70600	2.35E-05	1.66E-05	0.08558	0.06042
20000	0.70600	3.53E-05	2.49E-05	0.12836	0.09062
10000	0.70000	7.00E-05	4.90E-05	0.25455	0.17818
9000	0.69500	7.72E-05	5.37E-05	0.28081	0.19516
8000	0.69300	8.66E-05	6.00E-05	0.31500	0.21830
7000	0.69200	9.89E-05	6.84E-05	0.35948	0.24876
6000	0.68900	1.15E-04	7.91E-05	0.41758	0.28771
5000	0.68600	1.37E-04	9.41E-05	0.49891	0.34225
4000	0.68200	1.71E-04	1.16E-04	0.62000	0.42284
3000	0.67600	2.25E-04	1.52E-04	0.81939	0.55391
2000	0.66700	3.34E-04	2.22E-04	1.21273	0.80889
1000	0.61400	6.14E-04	3.77E-04	2.23273	1.37089
900	0.58900	6.54E-04	3.85E-04	2.37980	1.40170
800	0.56700	7.09E-04	4.02E-04	2.57727	1.46131
700	0.55900	7.99E-04	4.46E-04	2.90390	1.62328
600	0.54800	9.13E-04	5.01E-04	3.32121	1.82002

(Contd.)

Table 12.1 (*Continued*)

External resistance (Ω)	Voltage (V)	Current (A)	Power (W)	Current density (A/m^3)	Power density (W/m^3)
500	0.52800	1.06E-03	5.58E-04	3.84000	2.02752
400	0.51100	1.28E-03	6.53E-04	4.64545	2.37383
300	0.48400	1.61E-03	7.81E-04	5.86667	2.83947
200	0.45900	2.30E-03	1.05E-03	8.34545	3.83056
100	0.36500	3.65E-03	1.33E-03	13.27273	4.84455
90	0.31000	3.44E-03	1.07E-03	12.52525	3.88283
80	0.27800	3.48E-03	9.66E-04	12.63636	3.51291
70	0.25500	3.64E-03	9.29E-04	13.24675	3.37792
60	0.23000	3.83E-03	8.82E-04	13.93939	3.20606
50	0.20500	4.10E-03	8.41E-04	14.90909	3.05636
40	0.17400	4.35E-03	7.57E-04	15.81818	2.75236
30	0.13600	4.53E-03	6.17E-04	16.48485	2.24194
20	0.10400	5.20E-03	5.41E-04	18.90909	1.96655
10	0.06000	6.00E-03	3.60E-04	21.81818	1.30909
9	0.04900	5.44E-03	2.67E-04	19.79798	0.97010
8	0.04200	5.25E-03	2.21E-04	19.09091	0.80182
7	0.03700	5.29E-03	1.96E-04	19.22078	0.71117
6	0.03200	5.33E-03	1.71E-04	19.39394	0.62061
5	0.02700	5.40E-03	1.46E-04	19.63636	0.53018
4	0.02300	5.75E-03	1.32E-04	20.90909	0.48091
3	0.01800	6.00E-03	1.08E-04	21.81818	0.39273
2	0.01400	7.00E-03	9.80E-05	25.45455	0.35636
1	0.01000	1.00E-02	1.00E-04	36.36364	0.36364

Open-circuit voltage = 0.7503 V (taken before attaching resistance)

Theoretical value = 1.103 V

$$\text{Percentage error} = \frac{1.103 - 0.7503}{1.103} \times 100 = 31.98\%$$

12.6.2 Sample Calculations

$R = 10,000 \, \Omega, \, V = 0.70 \, V$

$$I = \frac{V}{R} = \frac{0.70}{10,000} = 7.0 \times 10^{-5} \, A$$

Power, $P = V \times I = (0.70 \times 7 \times 10^{-5}) \, W$

$$= 4.9 \times 10^{-5} \, W$$

$$\text{Current density } (I_d) = \frac{V}{R \times V_{\text{anode}}} = \frac{7.0 \times 10^{-5} \text{A}}{(275 \times 10^{-6})}$$

$$= 0.2545 \text{ A/m}^3$$

$$\text{Power density } (P_d) = \frac{V \times I}{v} = \frac{4.9 \times 10^{-5}}{275 \times 10^{-6}}$$

$$= 0.178 \text{ W/m}^3$$

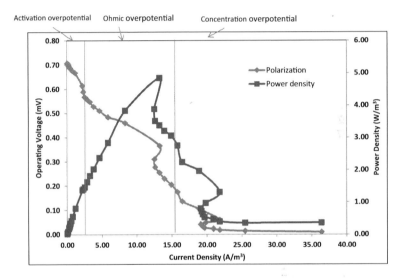

Figure 12.5　Polarization and power density curve.

Maximum power density $= 4.8445 \text{ W/m}^3$

At operating voltage $= 0.365 \text{ V}$

12.7 Discussion

12.7.1 Chemical Oxygen Demand

Chemical oxygen demand (COD) is the measurement of oxygen required to oxidize soluble and particulate organic matter in water. It is an important water-quality parameter. Higher COD level means a greater amount of oxidizable organic materials in the sample, which will reduce the dissolved oxygen (DO) level.

The method involves using a strong oxidizing agent $K_2Cr_2O_7$ to oxidize the organic matter in solution to CO_2 and H_2O under acidic conditions. Simultaneously, $Cr_2O_7^{2-}$ gets reduced to Cr^{3+} (green), and the concentration of Cr^{3+} is measured spectrophotometrically. The spectrometer only detects COD in the range of 0–1500 mg/L. Hence, we dilute the sample five times to get proper readings. The amount of oxygen required is calculated from the quantity of chemical oxidants consumed.

$$K_2Cr_2O_7 + H_2SO_4 \rightarrow K_2SO_4 + Cr_2(SO_4)_3 + 4H_2O + 3\,[O]$$

Apparatus: COD digester (HACH DRB 200)

Portable spectrophotometer (HACH DR2800)

Reagents: Distilled water

Solution 1: Mercuric sulfate (0.25 mL)

Solution 2: $\left.\begin{array}{l} k_2Cr_2O_7 \\ H_2SO_4 \end{array}\right\}$ (2.80 ml)

12.7.1.1 Procedure

(1) To the COD vials, 0.25 mL of solution 1 and 2.80 mL of solution 2 are added.
(2) Then 2 mL of the sample is added.
(3) The contents are mixed, and the COD vials are kept in the COD digester and heat is applied ($150°C$ to the vials and is refluxed for 2 h).
(4) After 2 h, the COD vials are carefully removed, and the COD is observed using HACH COD spectrophotometer.

$$\Delta COD = \text{Initial COD} - \text{Final COD}$$

$$= (3060 - 902.5)\,\text{mg/L}$$

$$= 2157.5\,\text{mg/L}$$

$$\text{COD removal efficiency} = \left(\frac{COD_i - COD_f}{COD_i} \right) \times 100$$

$$= 70.50654\%$$

$$\approx 70.51\%$$

COD of the samples from MFC at different time intervals are shown in Table 12.2. Figure 12.6 shows the COD degradation profile of the sample in MFC.

Table 12.2   COD of the samples at different intervals from MFC

Time (h)	COD (mg/L)
0	3060
12	2410
24	1347
36	902.5

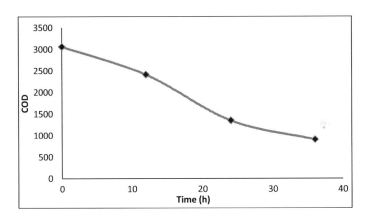

Figure 12.6   COD degradation profile in the MFC.

12.7.2 Columbic Efficiency

Columbic efficiency (Faraday efficiency) describes the efficiency with which charges (electrons) are transferred in a system facilitating an electrochemical reaction. From Eq. 12.9,

$$c_E = \frac{\text{Total charge coming out as output}}{\text{Total charge transferred by substrate (input)}}$$

$$C_E = \frac{M \int_0^{t_b} I\, dt}{F\, b\, V_{An}\, \Delta COD}$$

where $b = 4$ electrons from O_2, $M = 32$ g/g mol (mass of oxygen), $\int_0^{t_b} I\, dt$ is the current measured at time t_b, ΔCOD is the change in COD, V_{An} is the working volume of the anode chamber, and t_b is the batch time in s.

From the data obtained,

$It_b = 1388.86$ As, $F = 96500$ C, $V_{An} = 0.275$ L,

$\Delta COD = 2.157$ g/L

$$C_E = \frac{8 I t_b}{F V_{An} \Delta COD} = \frac{8 \times 1388.86}{96500 \times 0.275 \times 2.157}$$

$C_E = 6.8297\%$

Open-circuit voltage $= 0.7503$ V

Percentage error $= 3198\%$

Maximum power density $(P_d) = 4.8445$ W/m^3

At $R = 100$ Ω, $V = 0.365$ V, $I = 3.65$ mA

Chemical oxygen demand

$\Delta COD = 2157.5$ mg/L

COD removal efficiency $= 70.51\%$

Coulombic efficiency, $C_E = 6.83\%$

The open-circuit voltage we obtained is 0.7503 V. However, the theoretical value is 1.103 V. The difference in the result is due to the internal resistance of MFCs. The maximum power density is also very low. It has been demonstrated that the significant loss in MFC efficiency is due to the reactions occurring in the anode and cathode chambers.

It has also been speculated that the efficiency loss at the cathode is due to the low availability of protons. The concentration of protons is very low in the anodic chamber. That is why we have used an anion exchange membrane to avoid the movement of other cations to the cathodic chamber. However, a nanoporous membrane has been recently developed, which is kind of a nanoporous polymer filter and offers comparable power densities to PEM with greater durability. A porous membrane allows passive diffusion, thereby reducing the necessary power supplied to the MFC. Increasing the thickness of the anodes in MFCs with space between the electrodes can increase power production. The ohmic resistance decreases as the space between the electrodes is reduced, but the fact is that this does not increase the power output by MFCs.

Oxygen transfer through cathode adversely affects the power production at anode because in aerobic conditions, bacteria convert carbon compounds into CO_2 and H_2O, and due to this, proton and e^- are not released. Therefore, power can decrease with reduced electrode spacing despite improvement in ohmic resistance.

Voltage stabilizers can be used to stabilize the voltage at which maximum power is obtained. Further, voltage amplifiers and power amplifiers can be used to optimize the output from the MFCs. Energy harvested from MFCs can be used for devices such as remote sensors.

The age of the culture used in MFCs plays a major role both in wastewater treatment and in electricity generation. The culture should be in the log phase.

Further, the power from MFCs can be stored using a capacitor or any other suitable device, and the power can later be utilized in bulk since power output is low.

12.8 Conclusion

In the fuel cell polarization curve (plot of voltage versus current density), three distinct regions are noticeable (Fig. 12.1):

(1) At low current densities, the cell potential drops sharply because of activation polarization.

(2) At intermediate current densities, the cell potential drops linearly with current, clearly because of ohmic losses (i.e., cell resistance).

(3) At high current densities, the drop in cell potential departs from the linear relationship with the current density, due to more pronounced concentration polarization.

The coulombic efficiency of an MFC is the ratio of charge output to charge input. This is found to be 6.83% in the present experimental study.

References

1. Das, D., *Microbial Fuel Cell: A Bioelectrochemical System that Converts Waste to Watts*, Capital Publishing Company Ltd., New Delhi, India and Springer, Switzerland, 2017.

2. Mohan, Y., Manoj Muthu Kumar, S., and Das, D., Electricity generation using microbial fuel cells, *International Journal of Hydrogen Energy*, **33**: 423–426, 2008.

3. Varanasi, J. L., Kumari, S., and Das, D., Improvement of energy recovery from water hyacinth by using integrated system, *International Journal of Hydrogen Energy*, **43**: 1303–1318, 2018.

Experiment 13

Biosorption Kinetics

Objective: To estimate the kinetics and isotherms of biosorption reaction using *Mangifera indica*

13.1 Purpose

To evaluate the biosorption kinetics of a biochemical reaction and estimate the adsorption isotherms

13.2 Theory

The phenomenon of adsorption plays an important role in a biochemical reaction. The process of adsorption of heavy metals on biological surfaces is referred to as biosorption. Technically, biosorption is defined as the "ability of biological materials to accumulate heavy metals from wastewater through metabolically mediated (by the use of ATP) or spontaneous physicochemical pathways of uptake (not at the cost of ATP), or as a property of certain types of inactive, non-living microbial biomass which bind and concentrate heavy metals from even very dilute aqueous

Biochemical Engineering: A Laboratory Manual
Debabrata Das and Debayan Das
Copyright © 2021 Jenny Stanford Publishing Pte. Ltd.
ISBN 978-981-4877-36-7 (Hardcover), 978-1-003-11105-4 (eBook)
www.jennystanford.com

solutions." Hence, biosorption may be termed an important bio-chemical process for the removal of heavy metals from any downstream processes such as industrial effluent and wastewater. Recently, the phenomenon of biosorption has also been used to remove heavy metals from groundwater. Researchers are in the continuous search of cheap biosorbents for the removal of heavy metals. The current experimental demonstration involves the biosorption of cadmium ions on dried mango leaves.

13.2.1 Kinetic Modeling

Information on the kinetics of solute biosorption is crucial to design effective biosorption systems and also to select optimum operating conditions for a full-scale batch biosorption system. In addition, biosorption kinetics is beneficial in elucidating the mechanism and potential rate-controlling steps involved in the process of biosorption of metal ions on the biosorbents. For the present case, biosorption kinetics of pseudo-first-order and second-order kinetics are considered. Lagergren's pseudo-first-order model is based on the assumption that the rate of biosorption is proportional to the number of free active sites on the biosorbent's surface of dried and crushed mango leaves. The pseudo-first-order kinetic model (Eq. 13.1) is expressed as follows:

$$\frac{dq_t}{dt} = k_1(q_e - q_t) \tag{13.1}$$

where q_t and q_e are the biosorption capacities (mg/g) at time t (h) and equilibrium, respectively; and k_1 is the rate constant of the pseudo-first-order adsorption (h^{-1}). The biosorption capacity q can be easily calculated from $q = (c_0 - c_e) V/m$, where m is the dry weight of the biosorbent, V is the volume of the solution, and c_0 and c_e are the initial and equilibrium concentrations of cadmium in the solution. Integration of Eq. 13.1 with the boundary conditions $t = 0$ to $t = t$ and $q_t = 0$ to $q_t = q_t$ gives the following nonlinear expression (Eq. 13.2):

$$q_t = q_e(1 - e^{-k_1 t}) \tag{13.2}$$

Equation 13.2 can also be written as

$$\log(q_e - q_t) = \log q_e - \frac{k_1}{2.303}t \tag{13.3}$$

The pseudo-second-order kinetic model assumes that the biosorption rate is controlled by chemical sorption and proportional to the second power of the available fraction of active sites. The pseudo-second-order model is expressed as follows:

$$\frac{dq_t}{dt} = k_2(q_e - q_t)^2 \tag{13.4}$$

where q_e and q_t are the biosorption capacities (mg/g) at equilibrium and at any time $t = t$ (h), and k_2 is the rate constant of pseudo-second-order biosorption model (g/mg h). After integration and applying boundary conditions $t = 0$ to $t = t$ and $q_t = 0$ to $q_t = q_t$, the integrated and nonlinear form of Eq. 13.4 becomes

$$q_t = \frac{t}{\frac{1}{k_2 q_e^2} + \frac{t}{q_e}} \tag{13.5}$$

Equation 13.5 may be rearranged as

$$\frac{t}{q_t} = \frac{1}{k_2 q_e^2} + \frac{t}{q_e} \tag{13.6}$$

13.2.2 Equilibrium Modeling

The equilibrium distribution of cadmium ions between the aqueous phase and dried mango leaves biomass was expressed in terms of a cadmium biosorption isotherm. The Langmuir and Freundlich isotherm models, which have been the most widely used models to analyze data for water and wastewater treatment applications, are used in the present work to analyze the experimental equilibrium data of cadmium biosorption. The Langmuir isotherm model is based on the following assumptions: (1) all the adsorption sites are identical, (2) each adsorption site can retain one molecule of adsorbate and consequently the adsorption is limited to monolayer coverage, (3) all sites are energetically and sterically independent of the adsorbed quantity, and (4) the adsorptive forces are similar to the forces in the chemical interaction. The Langmuir equation is expressed as follows:

$$q_e = \frac{q_{max}\, bc_e}{1 + bc_e} \tag{13.7}$$

where q_e is the adsorption capacity at equilibrium (mg/g), q_{max} is the maximum adsorption capacity, also called the saturated monolayer adsorption capacity (mg/g), c_e is the liquid phase concentration of adsorbate at equilibrium (mg/L), and b (L/mg) is the adsorption equilibrium constant (Langmuir constant), which is related to the adsorption energy and quantitatively reflects the affinity between the sorbent and the sorbate.

Equation 13.7 can be modified and rewritten as follows:

$$\frac{c_e}{q_e} = \frac{1}{q_{max}\, b} + \frac{c_e}{q_{max}} \tag{13.8}$$

The Freundlich model is an empirical equation that applies to nonideal adsorption equilibrium on heterogeneous surfaces and also to multilayer adsorption, suggesting that binding sites are not equivalent and/or independent. This model assumes the following: There is an infinite supply of unreacted adsorption sites; the stronger binding sites are occupied first; the binding strength decreases with the increasing degree of site occupation; and there is a logarithmic reduction in the affinity between solute and adsorbent during surface coverage. The Freundlich isotherm expression is as follows:

$$q_e = k_F c_e^{1/n_F} \tag{13.9}$$

where k_F [(mg/g)(mg/L)]$^{-1}$ is a constant indicative of the relative adsorption capacity of the adsorbent and n_F is the heterogeneity factor, and its reciprocal indicates the intensity of adsorption. Equation 13.9 can be rewritten as follows:

$$\log q_e = \log k_F + \frac{1}{n_F} \log c_e \tag{13.10}$$

13.3 Apparatus and Chemicals Required

- Benchtop shaking incubator
- Cotton for plugging

- Oven for drying *Mangifera indica* (mango) leaves
- Mixer grinder for crushing the dried mango leaves into fine powder
- Cadmium nitrate
- Double-distilled water
- Spectroquant–cadmium test kit (Fig. 13.1)
- Sample collecting falcon tubes
- Stopwatch
- Whatman Grade no. 1 filter
- Test tubes for analysis

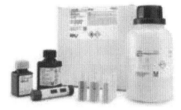

Figure 13.1   Spectroquant–cadmium test kit.

13.4 Methodology

13.4.1 Experimental Procedure for Calculating the Reaction Kinetics

(1) Cadmium nitrate solution of concentration 0.1 mg/L is prepared and distributed in 10 separate 100 mL conical flasks.

(2) Accurately weighed amounts of biomass (0.2 g) were added to a set of 10 glass flasks containing 50 mL of cadmium solution.

(3) The pH was adjusted to 5 using 0.1 N HCL and 0.1 N NaOH.

(4) The conical flasks are labelled for various times: 0 min, 5 min, 10 min, 20 min, 30 min, 40 min, 50 min, 60 min, 70 min, and 80 min.

(5) The conical flasks, except the one with 0 min label, are then inserted into the benchtop shaking incubator and the stopwatch is switched on.

(6) Shaking takes place for the required amount of time as mentioned in Step 3.

(7) Immediately after completion, the conical flasks are taken out and filtered using a Whatman Grade no. 1 filter paper.

(8) The filtered solution is then taken for analysis in the Spectroquant–cadmium test kit.

(9) The Spectroquant test kit consists of three reagents that need to be added. In a test tube, 1 mL of the first reagent, 10 mL of the filtered solution, 0.2 mL of the second reagent, and 1 level green microspoon of reagent 3 are added. The solution is then mixed and left to stand for 2 min. A part of this mixed solution is filled into a cell and inserted in the photometer for acquiring the concentration of cadmium. Note that the measured concentration refers to the cadmium concentration after biosorption (c_e).

13.4.2 Experimental Procedure for Estimating Isotherm Model

(1) Cadmium nitrate solutions corresponding to different concentrations—0.1 mg/L, 0.15 mg/L, 0.2 mg/L, 0.25 mg/L, and 0.3 mg/L—are taken in five separate conical flasks.

(2) To each conical flask containing 50 mL of cadmium nitrate solution, 0.4 g dried and crushed mango leaf powder is added.

(3) The pH is maintained by adding 0.1 N HCL and 0.1 N NaOH.

(4) The conical flasks were plugged and then kept in the incubator at a temperature of $25^{\circ}C$ for a period of 2 h in order to achieve the equilibrium.

(5) After 2 h, the flasks were taken out and the solutions were filtered using a Whatman Grade no. 1 filter paper.

(6) The filtered solutions were then taken for analysis in Spectroquant as described in the last step of Section 13.4.1.

13.5 Observation

After acquiring the value of equilibrium concentration from Spectroquant, the following parameters are calculated (Table 13.1) based on the equations given in Section 13.2.

Table 13.1 Cadmium concentration profile after biosorption (for an initial cadmium concentration of 0.1 mg/L and an adsorbent dosage of 0.2 g at a temperature of 25°C)

Time (t) (min)	Final cadmium concentration (c_t) (mg/L)	Initial concentration (c_0) − Final concentration (c_t) (mg/L)	Biosorption capacity (q_t)	t/q_t	log ($q_e − q_t$)
0	0.08	0.02	0.005	0	−1.78915
5	0.065	0.035	0.00875	571.428	−1.90309
10	0.042	0.058	0.0145	689.655	−2.1707
20	0.03	0.07	0.0175	1142.857	−2.42597
30	0.022	0.078	0.0195	1538.461	−2.75696
40	0.018	0.082	0.0205	1951.219	−3.12494
50	0.015	0.085	0.02125	2352.941	—
60	0.015	0.085	0.02125	2823.529	—
70	0.015	0.085	0.02125	3294.117	—
80	0.015	0.085	0.02125	3764.705	—

13.5.1 Sample Calculations

The second column of Table 13.1 demonstrates the final cadmium concentration (c_t) after biosorption. Let us see the sample calculation for $t = 5$ min.

At $t = 5$ min, $c_t = 0.065$ mg/L, $c_0 = 0.1$ mg/L

Therefore, $c_0 − c_t = 0.035$ mg/L

Amount of cadmium uptake by the biosorbent (q_t):

$$\frac{c_0 − c_t}{m} \times v = \frac{0.035}{0.2} \times 0.05 = 0.00875 \text{ mg/g}$$

Again from Table 13.2,

$$c_0 − c_e = 0.2 \text{ mg/L} − 0.078 \text{ mg/L} = 0.122 \text{ mg/L}$$

$$q_e = \frac{c_0 − c_e}{m} \times v = \frac{0.122}{0.2} \times 0.05 = 0.03 \text{ mg/g}$$

$$\frac{c_e}{q_e} = \frac{0.078}{0.03} = 2.6$$

Table 13.2 Determination of the final cadmium concentration for various initial cadmium concentrations involving an adsorbent dosage of 0.4 g at a temperature of 25°C

c_0	c_e	$(c_0 - c_e)$	q_e	c_e/q_e	$\log c_e$	$\log q_e$
0.1	0.015	0.085	0.0214	0.7	−1.8	−1.67
0.15	0.043	0.107	0.0268	1.6	−1.3	−1.57
0.2	0.078	0.122	0.03	2.6	−1.1	−1.52
0.25	0.125	0.125	0.03125	4	−0.9	−1.5
0.3	0.165	0.135	0.034	4.88	−0.78	−1.47

From Eq. 13.6,

$$\frac{t}{q_t} = \frac{1}{k_2 q_e^2} + \frac{t}{q_e}$$

and from Fig. 13.3,

$$\text{slope} = \frac{1}{q_e} = 44.2$$

$$q_e = 0.0226 \text{ mg/g}$$

Again from the intercept $\dfrac{1}{k_2 q_e^2} = 199.5$, $k_2 = 9.79 \text{ min}^{-1}$

From Eq. 13.8,

$$\frac{c_e}{q_e} = \frac{1}{q_{max} b} + \frac{c_e}{q_{max}}$$

and from Fig. 13.4,

$$\text{slope} = \frac{1}{q_{max}} = 28.1$$

$$q_{max} = 0.035 \text{ mg/g}$$

$$\text{Intercept} = \frac{1}{q_{max} b} = 0.357$$

Therefore, $b = 78.68 \text{ L/mg}$

Again, from Eq. 13.10,

$$\log q_e = \log k_F + \frac{1}{n_F} \log c_e$$

From Fig. 13.5,

intercept $= \log k_F = -1.322$; therefore, $k_F = 0.047$ L/g.

Slope $= 0.188 = \frac{1}{n_F}$; therefore, $n_F = 5.3$.

13.6 Results and Discussion

From Table 13.1, it is clearly observed that there is a marked difference between the final cadmium concentration after time t (c_t) and the equilibrium concentration (c_e). The later refers to the concentration of cadmium ions after reaching the equilibrium time, which corresponds to 50 min, whereas the former refers to the cadmium concentration after time t (min). Hence, c_e corresponds to 0.015 mg/L.

For estimating the pseudo-first-order fit, Eq. 13.3 is used and a plot between log ($q_e - q_t$) and t results in a linear relationship with negative slope (Fig. 13.2). The slope of Eq. 13.3 corresponds to $-k_1/2.303$. The pseudo-first-order rate constant k_1 is calculated as 0.0764 L/min. Based on Eq. 13.3, the theoretical q_e is calculated as 0.0165 mg/g, whereas the experimental q_e is found to be 0.02125 mg/g. Therefore, there exists a difference of 22.35% between the theoretical and experimental q_e. In order to estimate the pseudo-second-order fit, Eq. 13.6 is implemented. A plot between t/q_t versus t results in a positive slope of magnitude $1/q_e$ and intercept of

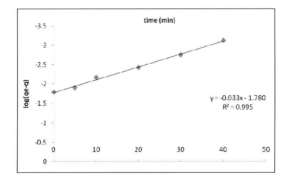

Figure 13.2 Pseudo-first-order kinetic plot based on Eq. 13.3.

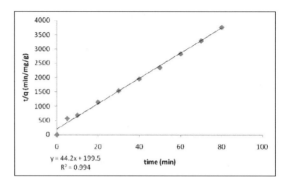

Figure 13.3 Pseudo-second-order kinetic plot based on Eq. 13.5.

$1/k_2 q_e^2$. Based on Eq. 13.6, the pseudo-second-order rate constant is estimated as 9.79 min^{-1} and the theoretical q_e is calculated as 0.0226 mg/g (Fig. 13.3). Thus, the difference between the theoretical and experimental q_e decreases to almost 5.97%. Hence, the pseudo-second-order rate equation results in a better fit than the pseudo-first-order fit.

The validity of the pseudo-second-order kinetic model signifies that the rate-limiting step may be chemical sorption involving valance forces either through sharing or exchange of electrons between heavy metal ions and the adsorbent. Based on theoretical considerations, the reaction of a divalent metal ion (M) binding to

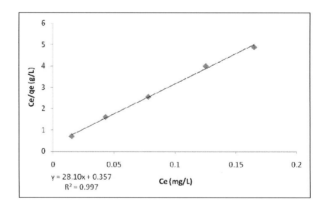

Figure 13.4 Langmuir adsorption isotherm plot based on Eq. 13.8.

two free binding sites B may be described. This indicates that the sorption rate would be proportional to the metal concentration and the square of the number of free sites. The better fit of the second-order model, therefore, indicates that a (1 : 2) binding stoichiometry applies, where one divalent metal binds to two monovalent binding sites.

Biosorption isotherms describe how adsorbate interacts with biosorbents, and equilibrium is established between the adsorbed metal ions on the biosorbent and the residual metal ions in the solution during the surface biosorption. Equilibrium isotherms are measured to determine the capacity of the biosorbent for metal ions. The equilibrium concentration along with the equilibrium uptake and all other necessary data are tabulated in Table 13.2.

The Langmuir adsorption isotherm fitted well as seen in Fig. 13.4 with $R^2 > 0.99$. The constants q_{max} and b are easily calculated based on Eq. 13.8, which demonstrates the slope and intercept as $1/q_{max}$ and $1/(q_{max} b)$, respectively. The q_{max} value is estimated as 0.035 mg/g, whereas the value of "b" is evaluated as 78.68 L/mg. The Freundlich isotherm fitting had $R^2 < 0.99$, and the Freundlich parameters are calculated from Eq. 13.10. The Freundlich constants "n_F" and "K_f" are evaluated as 5.3 and 0.047 L/g, respectively (Fig. 13.5). Since the fitting of the experimental data with the Langmuir isotherm is better than the Freundlich isotherm, it is expected that monolayer coverage of adsorbate over a homogeneous

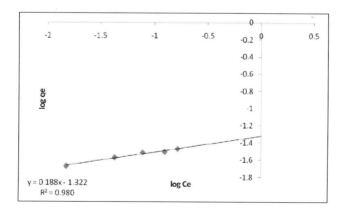

Figure 13.5 Freundlich adsorption isotherm plot based on Eq. 13.10.

adsorbent surface is occurring and the biosorption of each molecule on the surface has equal biosorption activation energy.

13.7 Conclusion

(1) Biosorption reaction that involves the adsorption of heavy metals on the surface of a sorbent follows second-order kinetics.
(2) Langmuir s model fitted the experimental equilibrium biosorption data, and the maximum total biosorption capacity was found to be 0.035 mg/g.

References

1. Cruz, C. C., Da Costa, A. C. A., Henriques, C. A., and Luna, A. S., Kinetic modeling and equilibrium studies during cadmium biosorption by dead *Sargassum* sp. Biomass, *Bioresource Technology*, **91**: 249–257, 2004.
2. Abdel-Aty, A. M., Ammar, N. S., Ghafar, H. H. A., and Ali, R. K., Biosorption of cadmium and lead from aqueous solution by fresh water alga *Anabaena sphaerica* biomass, *Journal of Advanced Research*, **4**: 367–374, 2013.
3. Ahmad, I., Akhtar, M. J., Jadoon, I. B. K., Imran, M., and Ali, S., Equilibrium modeling of cadmium biosorption from aqueous solution by compost, *Environmental Science and Pollution Research*, **24**: 5277–5284, 2017.
4. Harimawan, A., Haryani, G. S., and Setiadi, T., Equilibrium and kinetic modelling of cadmium (II) biosorption by dried biomass *Aphanothece* sp. from aqueous phase, *IOP Conference Series: Earth and Environmental Science*, **65**: 012018, 2017.
5. Camacho-Chab, J. C., Castañeda-Chávez, M. D. R., Chan-Bacab, M. J., Aguila-Ramírez, R. N., Galaviz-Villa, I., Bartolo-Pérez, P., and Ortega-Morales, B. O., Biosorption of cadmium by non-toxic extracellular polymeric substances (EPS) synthesized by bacteria from marine intertidal biofilms, *International Journal of Environmental Research and Public Health*, **15**: 314, 2018.
6. Satya, A., Harimawan, A., Haryani, G. S., Johir, M., Hasan, A., Vigneswaran, S., and Setiadi, T., Batch study of cadmium biosorption by carbon dioxide enriched *Aphanothece* sp. dried biomass, *Water*, **12**: 264, 2020.

Instrumentations

Spectrophotometer

Spectrophotometry is the quantitative measurement of the reflection or transmission properties of a material as a function of wavelength. It was first invented by Arnold O. Beckman in 1940. The most common spectrophotometric measurement is performed by a UV-VIS spectrophotometer, which uses light over the ultraviolet range (185–400 nm) and visible range (400–700 nm) of the electromagnetic radiation spectrum. Basic components of the instrument are light source, monochromator, sample holder, detector, and recorder. In a UV-VIS spectrophotometer, a light beam from a suitable source of ultraviolet and/or visible light passes through a monochromator prism. Light then passes the sample, and the transmitted light is measured at the detector. Light is absorbed by the liquid sample because it contains insoluble matter. Concentration of the sample is measured using the Beer–Lambert law, which states a linear relationship between absorbance and the sample concentration. The Beer–Lambert law can be expressed as

$$A = \varepsilon l c$$

where A is the absorbance, ε is the absorption coefficient, l is the optical path length, and c is the concentration of the sample.

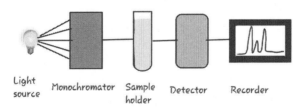

Light source   Monochromator   Sample holder   Detector   Recorder

Figure 1   Mechanism involved in spectrophotometry.

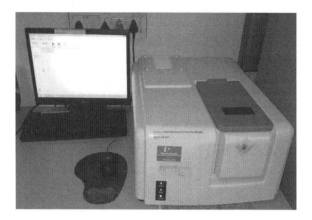

Figure 2 A UV-VIS spectrophotometer.

Nephelometer and Turbidimeter

Nephelometer and turbidimeter are usually used for the same purpose. They are used to measure the concentration of suspended particulates in a liquid–solid colloid. For turbidity measurement, a formazine suspension is prepared as a standard by mixing solutions of 10 g/L hydrazine sulfate and 100 g/L hexamethylenetetramine with ultrapure water. The suspension will be developed by keeping the solution for 24 h at 25°C. Mix and dilute 10.00 mL of stock standard suspension to 100 mL with water. The turbidity of this suspension is defined as 40 NTU. In turbidimetry, the intensity of light transmitted through the medium, the unscattered light, is measured. In nephelometry, the intensity of the scattered light is measured. The working mechanism is similar to that of a spectrophotometer. The components of a nephelometer are the same as those of a light spectrophotometer except that the detector is placed at a specific angle from the incident light. Since the amount of scattered light is far greater than the transmitted light in a turbid suspension, nephelometry offers higher sensitivity than turbidimetry. The unit is nephelometric turbidity units (NTU). A standard curve is prepared with respect to cell mass concentration and NTU unit. The usual conversion factor is 1 mg/l cell suspension = 3 NTU = 1 ppm.

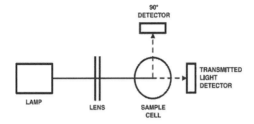

Figure 3   Mechanism involved in turbidimetry.

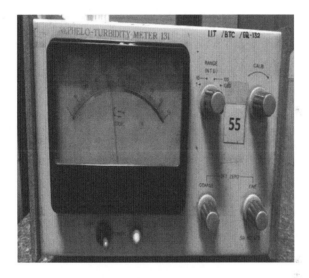

Figure 4   Nephelo-turbidimeter.

Table-Top Centrifuge

A centrifuge is an equipment used in downstream processing for solid–liquid, liquid–liquid separation based on density difference. The instrument was invented by English military engineer Benjamin Robins. A centrifuge works on the principle of centrifugation, where the acceleration at centripetal force causes denser substance to separate out along the radial direction at the bottom of the centrifuge tube. A higher density phase comes to the bottom of the tube, whereas a lighter one floats to the top. Centrifugation efficiency depends on density difference, rotational speed, residence time, operation pressure, and temperature.

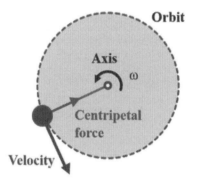

Figure 5   Mechanism involved in centrifugation.

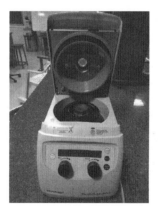

Figure 6   Table-top centrifuge.

Viscometer

A viscometer is an instrument used to measure the viscosity of a fluid. Viscometers are of six types: orifice viscometers, capillary viscometers, falling piston viscometers, rotational viscometers, falling ball viscometers, and vibrational viscometers.

Orifice Viscometers

An orifice viscometer usually consists of a cup with a hole through which fluid flows. Viscosity is measured by timing how long it takes the cup to empty. Orifice viscometers are easy to use manually.

Capillary Viscometers

A capillary viscometer is also known as a U-tube viscometer, which includes the Ostwald viscometer. It consists of a U-shaped glass tube with two bulbs (one higher and one lower). Fluid passes from the higher bulb to the lower bulb through a capillary, and viscosity is measured by timing how long the fluid takes to pass through the tube.

Falling Piston Viscometers

Falling piston viscometers are also called Norcross viscometers. They work by drawing the fluid being measured into the piston cylinder while the piston is raised; the time the piston takes to fall due to the resistance of the fluid is used to determine viscosity. It provides a long working life.

Rotational Viscometers

Rotational viscometers are suitable for both Newtonian and non-Newtonian fluids. These viscometers measure viscosity by immersing a rotating spindle in the fluid to be tested. The amount of power (torque) required to turn the spindle indicates the viscosity of the fluid, and because rotational viscometers do not use gravity to function, their measurements are based on the fluid's internal shear stress.

Falling Ball Viscometers

Falling ball viscometers are usually used for Newtonian fluids. Their working principle is similar to that of falling piston viscometers. A ball is dropped into a sample of the fluid being measured. The dimensions of the ball are already known, so viscosity is determined by timing how long the ball takes to fall through the fluid via gravity.

Vibrational Viscometers

Vibrational viscometers use a powered vibrating rod to measure viscosity. Viscosity of fluids is measured based on the vibration sensitivity of the fluid being tested.

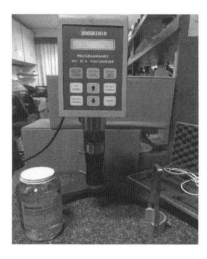

Figure 7 Laboratory-scale rotational viscometer.

pH Meter

A pH meter is a scientific instrument that measures the hydrogen ion activity in terms of acidity or basicity of a solution using a scale of 0–14. A pH meter is a potentiometric device that measures voltage as a response and changes it to the pH according to the Nernst equation. The electrodes or probes are inserted into the solution to be tested. Electrodes are rod-like structures usually made of glass, with a bulb containing the sensor at the bottom, which is specifically designed to be selective to hydrogen ion concentration. On immersion in the solution to be tested, hydrogen ions in the test solution exchange for other positively charged ions on the glass bulb, creating an electrochemical potential across the bulb. The electronic amplifier detects the difference in electrical potential between the two electrodes generated in the measurement and converts the potential difference to pH units. The magnitude of the

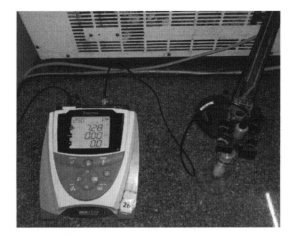

Figure 8   Potentiometric pH meter.

electrochemical potential across the glass bulb is linearly related to the pH according to the Nernst equation.

Incubator Shaker

An incubator shaker is a laboratory equipment used to mix, blend, or agitate substances in tubes or flasks by shaking them. It is widely used in the preparation of the microbial culture in conical flasks or test tubes. It is usually known as an orbital shaker, which has a circular shaking motion for mixing. This can be used for both

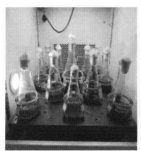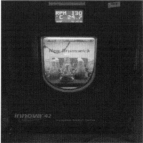

Figure 9   Incubator shaker (a) without illumination and (b) with illumination.

photobiological (with illumination) and non-photobiological growth of microbial cells (without illumination).

Laboratory-Scale Autoclave (Vertical)

An autoclave has the capability to use pressurized steam as the sterilization agent. The basic concept of an autoclave is to sterilize each item. The item may be liquid, glassware, or plasticware. These materials get sterilized when they come in direct contact with steam at a specific temperature (121°C) and pressure (15 psi) for a specific amount of time (15 min).

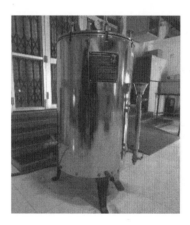

Figure 10   Autoclave.

Laminar Air Flow

A laminar flow cabinet is used to prevent the contamination of biological samples, or any particle-sensitive materials. It comprises a filter pad, a fan, and a high-efficiency particulate air (HEPA) filter. The fan sucks the air through the filter pad where dust is trapped. The sterile air flows into the working area where all culture preparation work can be carried out without the risk of contamination. Air is drawn through a HEPA filter and blown in a very smooth, laminar flow toward the user to maintain positive pressure inside the hood and contamination free.

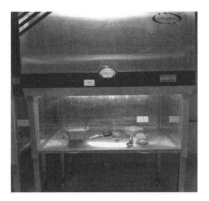

Figure 11   Laminar flow.

Microscope

A compound microscope is used to see the structure of the biological sample. It mainly consists of an objective lens, ocular lens, lens tube, stage, and reflector. An object placed on the stage is magnified through the objective lens. A magnified image can be visualized when the sample is focused through the ocular lens.

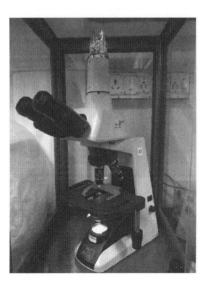

Figure 12   Compound microscope.

Appendices

A1 Gas Composition and Volatile Acid Analysis by Gas Chromatography (GC). SOP of Agilent GC

Theory: Gas chromatography is used for the quantitative estimation of mostly volatile samples. Measured amount of samples is injected in the injection port which is passed through the column and the detector with the help of carrier gas. The carrier gases are mostly inert, e.g. helium, argon, nitrogen, and hydrogen.

Sample

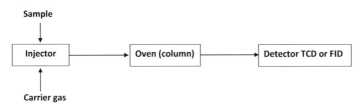

Carrier gas

Columns are either packed or capillary. Most packed column consists of a 1/8-inch-diameter tube of stainless steel, glass, etc., filled with stationary support materials ground in different sizes. The average length is 6 ft. The capillary tube inside diameter and length vary from 0.01 to 0.03 inch and 50–300 ft, respectively. They have no stationary phase packing materials. Instead, the stationary phase is coated onto the walls of the column. Such a column is called a wall-coated open tubular (WCOT) column.

A thermal conductivity detector (TCD) is mainly used for the analysis of gaseous samples. It is placed in the flowing steam of the effluent gas from the chromatographic column. The resistance of the wire depends on its temperature, which in turn is determined by the current flowing through the wire and by the rate at which heat is lost from the wire of thermal conductivity. The thermal conductivity of helium (and hydrogen) is very much greater than that of other gases. If helium is used as the carrier gas, the pressure of any solute around the wire will lower the thermal conductivity, raise the temperature of the wire, raise the resistance, and thus give rise to an electrical output signal that can be displayed on a recorder.

In the flame ionization detector (FID), the effluent from the column is mixed with hydrogen and oxygen for ignition. The hydrogen flame has very high resistance when only carrier gas (usually nitrogen) is flowing into it. When an organic compound enters the flame, its combustion produces ions that lower the flame's resistance, causing a current that is amplified by the electrometer and converted to a voltage. This voltage is read out by a recorder or by some digital device.

SOPs mean standard operating procedures (SOPs) for instruments. They include the standard protocol to be followed for the proper and efficient functioning of instruments during operation by students, faculty, lab technicians, and other researchers.

SOP for GC Agilent 7890A

To switch on the instrument

(1) Open the three cylinders (H_2, N_2, zero Air for FID and N_2 for TCD) and switch on the MCB for UPS.
(2) Switch on the MCB near the instrument and switch on all the switches (for GC, PC etc.)
(3) Switch on the PC and the GC (switch on front) and wait for the GC to be ready.
(4) Once the GC is ready, click on the **Agilent Online** icon and wait for the system to be ready.

To load the method for TCD

(1) From the dropdown menu of "Method," select **Tcd.m** for analyzing the gas samples.

(2) Once method is loaded, wait for the detectors to reach the "set" temperature.

(3) For TCD, the sample has to be loaded in the front inlet/port. However, to view the temperature and other settings, press the "Back Detector button (BACK DET)" on the machine.

(4) Enter the sample info from the Method → Sample Info. Enter your name (the subdirectory) where the data will be stored.

(5) Wait till the machine displays "READY FOR INJECTION" message on the left corner.

(6) Inject the sample and simultaneously press the START button on the machine.

(7) Wait till the analysis is done.

To load the method for FID

(1) For FID, select FID from the Method dropdown menu.

(2) For FID, the sample has to be injected in the back inlet/port, but to view the temperature and other settings, press the "Front Detector button (FRONT DET)" on the machine.

(3) Enter the sample info from the Method → Sample Info. Enter your name (the subdirectory) where the data will be stored.

(4) Wait till the machine displays "READY FOR INJECTION" message on the left corner.

(5) Inject the sample and simultaneously press the START button on the machine.

(6) Wait for the analysis to be completed.

The report will not be generated if the process is aborted.

To process the chromatograms

(1) The chromatograms can be accessed from the offline software.

(2) Double click on the **Agilent Offline** software and select your name (which is the subdirectory).

(3) From the subdirectory, double click on the file you want to view/edit. The chromatogram will open along with a table listing the different peaks detected along with its area.

(4) From the toolbox that opens above the chromatogram box, the undesired peaks can be cut.

(5) Save the changes to avail the desired data in the future.

To switch off the instrument

(1) After the analysis is completed, select the **COOLING method**, and wait till the temperature drops down to 50–60°C.
(2) Once the temperature drops down, switch off in the following sequence: close the software → shut down the PC → switch off the instrument switch → switch off the UPS → MCB → close the gas cylinders.

Troubleshoot

(1) Check whether all the gas flows are in the range or not.
(2) Check whether FID flame is ON during analysis.
(3) For online analysis, flush the sample at least for 5 min before injecting the sample.

A2 Analysis of Nonvolatile Organic Compounds by High-Performance Liquid Chromatography. SOP of Agilent HPLC

Principle

High-performance liquid chromatography (HPLC) is a highly sophisticated chromatographic technique used to separate compounds that are dissolved in a solution. Here the eluent is in the liquid phase. The principle of HPLC is that some molecules take longer than others to pass through a chromatography column, which is due to the affinity of the molecules with the mobile phase (liquid) and the stationary phase (solid). It is called HPLC due to high-pressure liquid in the mobile phase. Like GC, this also includes injector, column, and detector. Different detectors can be used, such as UV-VIS detector and refractive-index detector.

SOP for HPLC with RID

Agilent 1260 series

Operating steps:

(1) Connect the instrument to the stabilizer/UPS.

(2) Switch on the computer and then the instrument.

(3) There are four parts in the HPLC instrument: (i) degasser and pump, (ii) column compartment, (iii) MWD (UV-visible), and (iv) RID.

(4) Switch on all the four parts, and an orange-colored light will come. This means that the instrument is ON but not ready.

(5) Double click on the HPLC online software (Chemstation online).

(6) To start the program, go to HPLC online in the computer; 1–2 min will take to initialize.

(7) It will ask for the configuration upgrade; click No.
(If you want to change the configuration select yes → click on the auto configuration → OK. Select the IP Address → 192.168.254.11 → Click OK → ok.)

(8) The solvent bottle must be cleaned properly with water and finally must be rinsed with HPLC-grade solvents.

(9) Before you start, open the Black knob and allow the solvent to pass out without entering the column. This will not allow the air bubbles to pass through the column.
When you are sure that no bubble is there in the column,

(10) Click on the Instrument → System on.

(11) Open the purge method → Select flow 5 mL, pressure 200 bar by selecting 100% for each channel till all the bubbles come out from each flowline around 5 min.

(12) Set the flow rate to 0 mL/min.

(13) Close the Back knob.

(14) Using the HPLC Chemstation software, load the respective method for analyzing the sample.

(15) Now the solvent passes through the column.

(16) For RID → right click on the RID panel → select purge valve on and put it for 1 h.
Then close the purge valve and do the balancing.

(17) Before starting the analysis, the column must be equilibrated for at least 1 h or maximum 4 h with the solvent.

(18) Check the baseline for individual channels. If it is ok, then do the injection of sample.

(19) To inject the sample:

- Turn the injector knob to load.

- Insert the syringe into the needle port. You will feel tightness during the last 2–3 mm of travel as the needle passes through the needle seal and stops against the stator face.
- Load the sample.
- Leave the syringe in and turn to INJECT.

(20) After completion, the chromatogram can be accessed using the Chemstation offline software.

(21) Stop the flow.

(22) If buffer solution is used then clean the flow lines with 100% water.

(23) For doing that, first do the purging for 5 min and then set the flow rate to 1 mL/min for 30 min.

(24) Then flash the flowline with 1:1 (acetonitrile: water) or (methanol: water) at 1 mL/min flow rate.

(25) Then stop the flow and switch off the system.

(26) Click on the instrument off button.

(27) Close the Chemstation online software.

(28) Switch off the power button of the instrument.

A3 Metal Ions Present in the Sample by Atomic Absorption Spectrophotometer

Atomic absorption spectrophotometer (ASS) use the absorption of light to measure the concentration of gas phase atoms. A high voltage is passed between the cathode and anode, and the metal atoms are excited into producing light with a certain emission spectrum. The principle of atomic emission spectroscopy involves the examination of the wavelengths of photons discharged by atoms and molecules as they transit from a high-energy state to a low-energy state. It is an analytical technique that measures the concentrations of elements. Atomic absorption is so sensitive that it can measure down to parts per billion of a gram ($\mu g/dm^3$), i.e., ppb in a sample. The samples are to be injected in the soluble form. Solid samples are usually digested with the acidic solution for solubilization. The soluble sample is drawn in the flame of ASS by the process of ejector. The operating principle of the ejector is that the pressure energy in the motive fluid is converted to velocity energy by an adiabatic expansion in the converging/diverging nozzle. Due to the pressure drop of the motive fluid, it will create a low-pressure zone before the mixing chamber. In the case of ASS, the moving fluids are air and acetylene. The technique makes use of the wavelengths of light generated by the hollow cathode lamp (HCL) specifically absorbed by an element (like Cu, Ni, etc.). The concentration is monitored based on the Beer–Lambert law. Absorbance is directly proportional to the concentration of the analyte absorbed for the existing set of conditions. In analytical chemistry, AAS is a technique used mostly for determining the concentration of a particular metal element within a sample.

The Beer–Lambert law states that there is a linear relationship between the concentration and the absorbance of the solution, which enables the concentration of a solution to be calculated by measuring its absorbance. It can be expressed as

$$A = \varepsilon bc \qquad (A3.1)$$

where A is absorbance (no units), ε is the molar absorptivity with units of L/mol cm (formerly called the extinction coefficient), and b is the path length of the sample, usually expressed in cm.

Again

$$A = \frac{I}{I_0} \qquad (A3.2)$$

where I_0 is the intensity of light before absorption and I is that after absorption.

A4 Chemical Oxygen Demand (COD) Determination of the Waste Samples by Titrimetric Method

Theory

The basis for the chemical oxygen demand (COD) test is that nearly all organic compounds can be fully oxidized to carbon dioxide with a strong oxidizing agent under acidic conditions. The amount of oxygen required to oxidize an organic compound to carbon dioxide, ammonia, and water is given by

$$C_nH_aO_bN_c + \left(n + \frac{a}{4} - \frac{b}{2} - \frac{3}{4}c\right)O_2$$

$$\rightarrow nCO_2 + \left(\frac{a}{2} - \frac{3}{2}c\right)H_2O + cNH_3 \qquad (A4.1)$$

Potassium dichromate is a strong oxidizing agent under acidic conditions. (Acidity is usually achieved by the addition of sulfuric acid.) The reaction of potassium dichromate with organic compounds is given by

$$C_nH_aO_bN_c + dCr_2O_7^{2-} + (8d + c)H^+$$

$$\longrightarrow CO_2 + \frac{a + 8d - c}{2}H_2O + cNH_4^+ + 3dCr^{3-} \qquad (A4.2)$$

where $d = 2n/3 + a/6 - b/3 - c/2$. Most commonly, a 0.25 N solution of potassium dichromate is used for COD determination, although for samples with COD below 50 mg/L, a lower concentration of potassium dichromate is preferred.

In the process of oxidizing the organic substances found in the water sample, potassium dichromate is reduced (since in all redox reactions, one reagent is oxidized and the other is reduced), forming Cr^{3+}. The amount of Cr^{3+} is determined after oxidization is complete and is used as an indirect measure of the organic contents of the water sample.

Method

COD determination is a measurement of the oxygen equivalent of the portion of organic matter in a sample that is susceptible to oxidation by a strong chemical oxidant. Standard Methods (APHA, 1992) open reflux method was used.

A sample of 20 mL was diluted to 50 mL with distilled water and added with 0.4 g of mercuric sulfate and anti-bumping granules. The mixture was then refluxed for 2 h with 10 mL of standard potassium dichromate solution and 30 mL of sulfuric acid reagent. The sample was cooled down and diluted to 140 mL with distilled water. The sample was then titrated with 0.1 M ferrous ammonium sulfate using ferroin solution as indicator. The end point is a sharp color change from blue–green to reddish–brown. The amount of oxidizable organic matter, measured as oxygen equivalent, is proportional to the potassium dichromate used. The COD was calculated based on the formula as follows:

$$\text{COD (mg/L)} = \frac{8000\,(A-B)\,N}{\text{Sample volume (mL)}} \qquad \text{(A4.3)}$$

where A is the volume (mL) of ferrous ammonium sulfate used for the titration of blank, B is the volume (mL) of ferrous ammonium sulfate used for sample titration, and N is the normality of ferrous ammonium sulfate.

One molecule of ferrous ammonium sulfate (FAS) reacts with 8 g of oxygen to convert into ferric ions. The equivalent weight of FAS is equal to its molecular weight.

$$2\text{FeSO}_4 \cdot (\text{NH}_4)_2\text{SO}_4 + \text{H}_2\text{SO}_4 + (\text{O}) \rightarrow \text{Fe}_2(\text{SO}_4)_3 + \text{H}_2\text{O} \quad \text{(A4.4)}$$

$$\text{Amount of FAS consumed} = (A-B)\,\text{mL}\,\frac{1\,\text{L}}{1000\,\text{mL}}\,\frac{\text{Mole of FAS}}{\text{L}}$$

$$= \frac{(A-B)}{1000}\,\text{mole of FAS}$$

x mL sample requires $\dfrac{(A-B)}{1000}$ mole of FAS

1 L sample requires $\dfrac{(A-B)}{1000\,x}$ 1000 mole of FAS $= (A-B)$ mole of FAS

From Eq. A4.4, we get 1 mole of FAS reacts with 8 g of oxygen.

Therefore, $(A-B)$ mole of FAS react with $8000\,(A-B)$ mg of oxygen.

A5 Determination of Heat of Combustion by Bomb Calorimeter

Description

A Parr bomb calorimeter to accurately determine the heat of combustion of a sample of biomass.

Theory

Calorimetry is an important field of analytical chemistry that deals with accurately measuring heats of reaction and finds applications in fields ranging from nutritional analysis to explosive yield test for estimating the heats of combustion of fuels. Heat of combustion or calorific value of fuel is of particular importance in the field of biofuels to evaluate the energy content in the fuel. The heat of combustion (ΔH_{comb}) is the total energy released as heat when a substance undergoes complete oxidation in the presence of oxygen under standard conditions.

A hydrocarbon undergoes complete combustion in the presence of oxygen. The energy is released in the form of heat (since combustion is an exothermic reaction).

$$C_x H_y O_z \text{ (s)} + \frac{\left(2x + \frac{y}{2} - z\right)}{2} O_2 \text{ (g)} \rightarrow x CO_2 \text{ (g)} + y H_2 O \text{ (l)} \quad \text{(A5.1)}$$

Principle

A bomb calorimeter is a type of constant volume calorimeter that measures the heat of combustion of a fuel (preferably solids and sometimes liquid). A bomb calorimeter typically consists of a metal bomb designed to withstand heat and pressure, a large Dewar flask to hold the bomb and a known volume of water, a means of remotely igniting the sample (typically electrically through the use of a fuse wire), and a means of accurately measuring the temperature of water.

Initially, the bomb is filled with a known volume of compressed oxygen so that complete combustion occurs. Electrical energy is used to ignite the fuel. As the fuel is burned, it will heat up the surrounding air. The sealed bomb acts as a closed system, and the energy from the adiabatic combustion of a known mass of sample will heat the bomb calorimeter and the water a measurable amount. Through the use of a calibration sample of known combustion value (such as benzoic acid), the heat capacity of a calorimeter system can be determined allowing for calculation of the heat of combustion of a sample of known mass by the net temperature change and the heat capacities of the combined water calorimeter system.

Parts of a Bomb Calorimeter

(1) **Thermometer (inbuilt)**: Used to measure the temperature rise in water. It is highly sensitive.

(2) **Stirrer**: Maintains uniformity and homogeneity of temperature inside.

(3) **Insulating jacket**: Used for insulation so that no heat transfer between the calorimeter and its surrounding occurs (no heat loss from the calorimeter or no heat transfer in). It is important because of the combustion reaction.

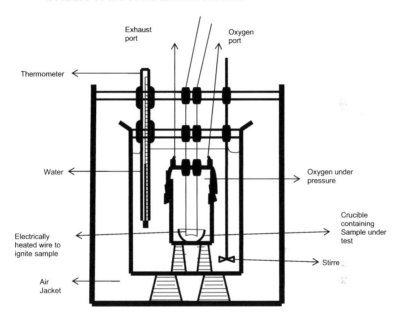

Figure A5.1 Schematic diagram of a bomb calorimeter.

(4) **Bomb**: Part where the whole combustion process occurs. It is made up of nickel and chromium alloy, which makes it resistant to corrosion and prevents explosion.

(5) **Crucible**: Something that is used to put the sample when it is exposed to high temperature. It is made up of heat-resistant materials.

(6) **Oxygen supply**: Provides oxygen to the part where combustion occurs.

(7) **Buckets**: It is the container for the flask in which water is put.
(8) **Ignition coil and wires**: Used for ignition of the combustion (burning of the sample in the presence of oxygen).

Spiking

If we take a partially combustible fuel or a fuel with very low calorific value or a fuel whose pure form is available in very low quantity for the measurement of calorific value, we need to completely burn it. For that the fuel is mixed with a known amount of benzoic acid whose calorific value is already known to the system. The mixture is then combusted, and the system automatically subtracts the energy content of benzoic acid giving only the energy content of the desired fuel.

Equipment used

Parr 6100 calorimeter

Oxygen cylinder

Cylinder pressure = 123 psi

Inlet pressure = 25 psi

Materials required:

(1) Biomass (pre-weighted): 0.507 g
(2) Distilled water: 2 L
(3) Benzoic acid pellet: 1 g
(4) Cotton thread

Procedure

(1) The weighed sample is placed in the provided crucible. An ignition thread of known length is carefully tied to the electrode arrangement provided in the bomb to ignite the sample, and the entire contents are sealed in the bombs.
(2) A known volume of compressed oxygen is filled into the bomb using leak-proof tubing.

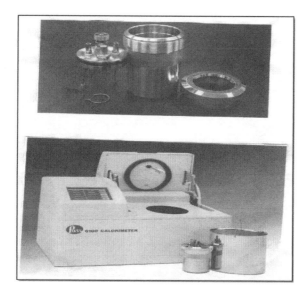

Figure A5.2   Parr bomb calorimeter.

(3) The steel bucket is carefully cleaned and filled with 2 L of distilled water and placed in the bomb calorimeter.

(4) The bomb is then carefully placed in the distilled water. It is to be ensured that the temperature probe and the stirrer are in appropriate position before closing the lid.

(5) Through the software, the ignition is started, and the combustion takes place in the device.

Observation

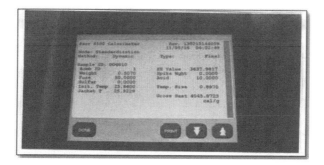

Result

Table A5.1   Calorific values of different samples

Sl. No	Name of the sample	Temperature rises (°C)	Heat of combustion (H_{comb}) (cal/g)
1.	Benzoic acid (C_6H_5COOH)	1.4014	6310.3
2.	Algal biomass (dried)	0.8970	4045.87

Reported calorific value of benzoic acid $= 6250$ cal/g

Experimental calorific value of benzoic acid $= 6310.3$ cal/g

$$\text{Percentage error} = \frac{6310.3 - 6250}{6250} \times 100 = 0.96\%$$

Discussion

A bomb calorimeter is an instrument that can efficiently measure the calorific value/heat of combustion of the fuel. The higher heating value (HHV) and the lower heating value (LHV) can be both measured using a bomb calorimeter. For measuring the HHV, all the combustion products are brought down to the pre-combustion condition so that all the water vapor condenses and the latent heat of atoms is present. To avoid the release of SO_2 and NO_x, around 1 mL of water in added to the bomb, which absorbs the acidic gases.

For determining the LHV, vaporization is added to the heat of combustion. The combustion products are kept in vapor. By knowing any one of the above, the other can be calculated using the formula mentioned in the theory.

Both the heating values can be related as:

$$HHV = LHV + H_v \left(\frac{n_{H_{2}0,\,out}}{n_{fuel,\,in}} \right) \tag{A5.2}$$

$H_v =$ heat of vaporization of water.

Due to combustion reactions of the fuel, carbon dioxide, sulfur dioxide, and nitrogen oxides are formed providing sulfur and nitrogen.

Source of error

(1) Incorrect measurement of weight of biomass or water.

(2) If an unknown sample is taken and the composition contains Cl_2 or SO_4, then it gets added in the acid content or may be the calorific value.

(3) If the sample is not completely dried and moisture is left, it evaporates on combustion, goes to the latent heat of vaporization, and gets either consumed or added to the calorific value.

A6 SOP for Software in PC Connected with Biojenik Engineering Fermenter

(1) First switch ON the electric switch for power connection of the fermenter control panel, compressor, chiller, and computer. Connect all the probes with the control panel and calibrate as mentioned in another SOP of the fermenter. (Please contact Professor Debabrata Das for Log In password of the computer.)

(2) Then open the software by double clicking on the software logo named "SIMATIC winC . . ."

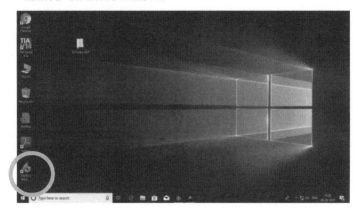

(3) Two windows will open: "WinCC Explorer . . ." and "WinCC Runtime." "WinCC Explorer . . ." will be used for changing any kind of setting. "WinCC Runtime" will be used for fermenter

operation. DO NOT CHANGE ANYTHING IN THE "WinCC Explorer . . ."

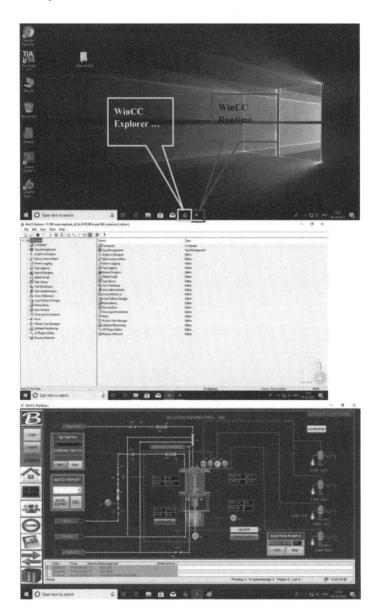

(4) Go to the "WinCC Runtime" windows where the schematic diagram of the system is shown. Log In by clicking on the Login button (upper left corner) using the following username and password:
Username: biojenik
Password: biojenik

(5) All the process parameters can be controlled after logging in the software. The controlled buttons for several parameters are shown in the picture.

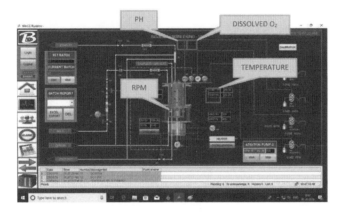

For example, for controlling agitation speed (rpm), click "M" as shown in the picture and then click "ON."

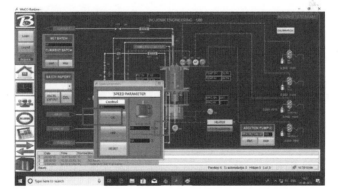

Agitation speed (rpm) can be changed by changing the set value (STIRC SV).

Note: There are two values shown in a tubular form. The upper value indicates the set value (SV) and the lower one for process actual value (AV).

Similarly, other parameters can be controlled.

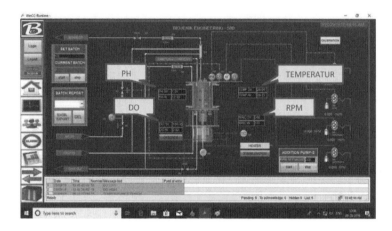

(6) For sterilization of the fermenter, click the "STERILIZATION" button and ON the sterilization process as shown in the picture.

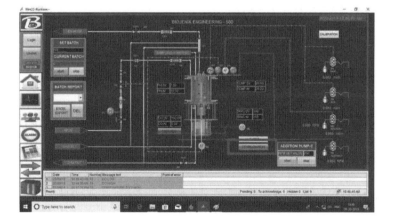

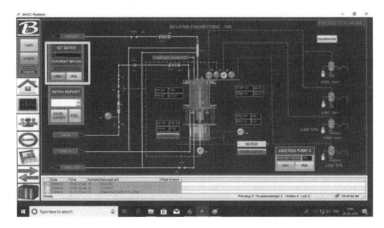

(7) Acid and base pump can be calibrated by clicking on the "CALIBRATION" button (top right corner).

(8) Once the operation is started, you need to set the batch number for data recording (if you wish). To set the batch number, write batch number in "SET BATCH" → enter → "START."

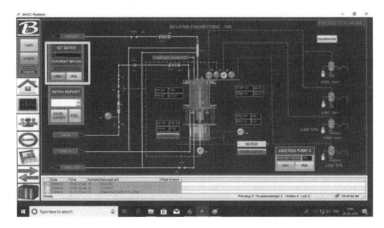

(9) After the completion of the batch, a report can be generated in an MS EXCEL SHEET. Write the batch number in "BATCH REPORT" → enter → click "EXCEL REPORT."

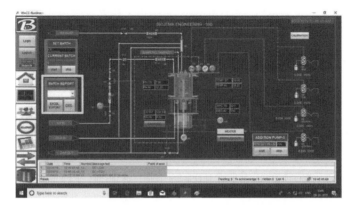

(10) Shut down of the software and the process: First turn OFF the control mode for all process parameters (PH, DO, RPM, TEMPERATURE).

For example, for RPM

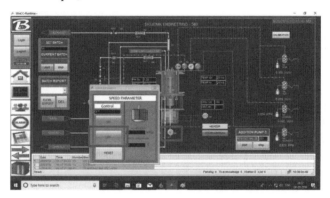

If feed pumps are ON, then turn OFF the same. "Logout" of the software by clicking on the Logout button (top left corner).

Close "WinCC Runtime" first, then "WinCC Explorer . . ." and shutdown the computer. Subsequently, turn OFF the control panel, compressor, and chiller.

Probable Questions

(1) What information you get from the layout of the fermenter?
(2) Discuss the purpose of the non-return valve of the fermenter.
(3) What do you mean by in vitro and in situ sterilization?
(4) Where is the condenser located in the fermenter?
(5) What is the purpose of air filter at the exhaust air line?
(6) How will you draw the sample from the fermenter?
(7) What is the purpose of the mechanical seal in the fermenter?
(8) What is the special feature of the sterilizable pH probe as compared to the ordinary pH probe?
(9) How is the temperature of the fermenter monitored?
(10) Define the activity of the enzyme. How will you express the same?
(11) Write the mathematical expression on the correlation between substrate concentration and time of enzymatic reaction.
(12) Write the limitations of the Michaelis–Menten equation.
(13) How will you find out K_m, v_{max}, and $k_a a_m$ of the immobilized enzymatic reaction?
(14) What is the significance of the value of K_m of an enzyme?
(15) Write the difference of Lineweaver–Burk plots of free and immobilized enzymatic reaction.
(16) Write the Monod equation for the cell growth kinetics. What do you mean by growth-limiting substrate?
(17) Write the limitations of the Monod equation for the cell growth kinetics?
(18) Write down the Pirt equation. What is the significance of maintenance coefficient?
(19) What do you mean by growth-associated and non-growth-associated products? Give examples.
(20) What are the units of growth-associated and non-growth-associated coefficients?

(21) Discuss the effect of fungal mycelium on yeast bacterial fermentation.

(22) Name at least two different analytical methods for the determination of glucose concentration in the fermentation broth.

(23) Differentiate between doubling time and generation time of the microbial cell.

(24) Name two antifoam agents used in the fermentation process.

(25) How is the doubling time of bacteria, yeast, and microalgae varied from each other?

(26) What is the unit of $k_L a$? Name at least two methods for the determination of $k_L a$.

(27) What do you mean by respiratory quotient? Discuss the importance of this parameter in Baker's yeast fermentation.

(28) What parameters influence the value of $k_L a$?

(29) Discuss the use of ocular lenses and stage for the determination of the diameter of microbial cell.

(30) Write the advantages of using a rotameter to find out the gas flow rate in comparison to a gas flow meter.

(31) Differentiate among η_o, η_α, and η of air filter.

(32) Write the advantages of using glass wool fiber for air sterilization.

(33) How do you calculate the power drawn by the agitator? Name different types of agitators used in a fermenter.

(34) What do you mean by the agitator Reynolds number?

(35) Write the reasons for using carboxy methyl cellulose (CMC) for the experimental study on mixing time determination.

(36) What are the drawbacks of the mixing time determination experiment?

(37) What is the purpose of the determination of cell density?

(38) What are the usual sizes of bacteria, yeast, and microalgae?

(39) What do you mean by the death rate constant of a microbial cell? How is it related with the decimal reduction time?

(40) Why UV rays were used for the kill curve experiment? Write some uses of this experimental study.

(41) Write the kinetic parameters that can be determined in the fermentation process like biohydrogen fermentation.

(42) What do you mean by a chemostat? Explain the major drawbacks of a chemostat.

(43) What is the special feature of the batch fermentation process in comparison to chemostat?

(44) Discuss the advantages of a chemostat in comparison to batch process.

(45) What is the correlation among μ_{max}, D_{max}, and $D_{washout}$?

(46) How will you overcome the cell washout problem of a chemostat?

(47) Write the principles used in the operation of a peristaltic pump. Why is this pump used in the biochemical industry? Name at least two companies manufacturing this pump.

(48) What is the significance of the polarization curve?

(49) Define Coulombic efficiency of a microbial fuel cell.

(50) Differentiate between adsorption and absorption with examples.

(51) What do you mean by Langmuir and Freundlich isotherms?

(52) Discuss the basic principles involved in gas chromatography (GC) and high-performance liquid chromatography (HPLC). Write the applications of these techniques.

(53) Name the detectors used in GC and HPLC.

(54) What are the different types of columns available in GC?

(55) Write the principle of the ejector. How is it used in an atomic absorption spectrophotometer?

(56) What do you mean by hollow cathode lamp?

(57) Discuss the principles of the bomb calorimeter.

(58) What do you mean by higher and lower heating values of a fuel?

(59) Explain the Beer–Lambert law.

(60) What do you mean by SOPs of the instrument?

(61) Name the different makes of the following:

    (a) Sterilizable pH probe

    (b) Controlled fermenter

    (c) DO probe

    (d) Gas flow meter

    (e) Centrifuge

Index